White Pajamas

17 Days at an A

KUNAL GUPTA

SPARK

Introduction
Stepping into stillness

I had been feeling called to go for a few months, yet every time I reached out to the hospital, they had no availability. Every few days, I sent them an email asking if anyone had canceled and, if a spot opened up, could they let me know? They kindly acknowledged my email each time and went on to remind me that people pay deposits months, even years in advance, and rarely cancel their bookings.

Nevertheless, being used to successful negotiations in business and getting what I want, I continued to believe that somehow this would happen. *And soon.*

Then after a few weeks of waiting, the fateful email arrived. A spot had just opened up, due to an unexpected cancelation. I responded immediately, telling myself I'd figure out the logistics of traveling to India from where I was currently staying in Australia.

I was sitting in an apartment hotel in Surry Hills, a suburb of Sydney, not too far from the central business district and tourist areas. I had arrived in Australia on a whim the previous week, flying across the world from Toronto during the Christmas holidays after my sister had jokingly challenged me to book a flight anywhere in the world within the week. I said I was craving some sun, and, as younger sisters often do, she thought of the farthest place on the planet I could go. Challenge accepted, I was on a plane a few hours later. Upon arriving in Australia, my spirits lifted instantly. Everyone looked as if they were going to or coming from the gym or the beach. Everyone appeared to be in a good mood. The sun shone brightly. I wore shorts every day, while my sister back home in Canada was shoveling snow off her front porch and wearing layer upon layer to stay warm.

While the Aussie culture and environment provided a temporary relief to my winter blues, something deeper was going on within me that would need to be addressed. That's why I'd been researching Ayurvedic hospitals in India, where I could go for an extended detox treatment program that I had heard about. During my yoga teacher training, which I did five years previously in New York City, we had a weekend introduction to yoga's "sister science," Ayurveda. I was immediately fascinated by it.

Ayurveda, a Sanskrit term, from *āyus* ("life") and *veda* ("sacred knowledge"), translates into English as the "study of life," is one of the world's oldest medical systems, dating back over 5,000 years. Throughout history, Ayurveda has been a significant part of South Asian culture and medical practice. Its influence is not confined to India, though; it has also shaped the development of other forms of medicine, such as Traditional Chinese Medicine, Unani Tibb medicine (practiced in South and Central Asia), and more.

The wisdom of Ayurveda was initially passed from sages to disciples orally, through verses known as *slokas* that were memorized and recited. This knowledge was eventually compiled and recorded in the Vedas, the ancient sacred texts of India. Ayurveda's foundational texts were written between 1500 BCE and 500 AD. These texts elaborate on various aspects of Ayurveda, including philosophy, preventive healthcare, the treatment of various ailments using dietary, lifestyle, and herbal interventions, and even surgical techniques.

Ayurveda is based on the premise that the universe comprises five elements—space, air, fire, water, and earth—which exist in every living being in varying proportions. Because of this, our human experience is inherently tied to the nature around us; there's a saying that goes, "we are microcosms of the macrocosm," to explain how the environment affects our individual bodies, and vice versa. These elements combine to form the three *doshas*, or life forces, that serve biological functions in the human body and in nature: *vata* (space and air), *pitta* (fire and water), and *kapha* (water and earth). Note that "dosha" is not to be confused with "dosa," the South Indian version of a tasty crepe. Ayurveda suggests that one's health is determined by maintaining the right balance of the doshas and elements, and an excess, deficiency, or malfunction of one or more doshas leads to disease.

Living in a state of "balance" in Ayurveda does not mean having an equal amount of all three doshas, however. Rather, balance means living in alignment with one's inherent constitution. Determining your constitution requires a careful analysis of many factors, including separating constitution from the current disease state. Someone's constitution might be dominant in one or more doshas, for example *vata* and *pitta*, but another dosha, like *kapha*, is weak, creating imbalance.

While many resources, such as "dosha quizzes," exist online, I've learned that it's best to work with a qualified practitioner to determine one's constitution and how to best support your unique state of balance.

All this is to say: Ayurveda is personalized medicine. It recognizes that each of us is unique, meaning that what my body needs to be healthy may be different from what your body needs. Maintaining balance requires attention to the health of the body, mind, and spirit, as well as taking into account the needs of our "season" of life—the season of nature, our age, and our current responsibilities.

When confronting any imbalance, the first step in Ayurveda is to try to restore the proportions and functions of the doshas within the system. This might include dietary changes or digestive support with herbal medicine, changes in one's schedule or daily routine, yoga or fitness protocols, and so on.

Depending on the severity and duration of the imbalance, it might take weeks, months, or years to see a full recovery—depending in part on a person's compliance with the suggestions. If an imbalance is too intense or long-term to respond to these at-home techniques, a more aggressive detoxification protocol, known as panchakarma, may be appropriate. Meaning "five actions," panchakarma comprises five detox treatments that maybe used in any combination, which is determined by a person's particular imbalances or disease. This also includes preparatory treatments and a period of reintegration to rebuild the body after cleansing.

While I dabbled in Ayurvedic routines after my yoga teacher training, I didn't know about panchakarma until a friend shared his experience with me. Martin was fifty-four years old but looked thirty-four—except for his full head of white hair. Martin and I met on a shamanic retreat together in the south of Portugal a year and a half before I booked my trip to India. Over lunch one day, he told me that he and his wife go for an Ayurveda detox each year in India. My memories of learning about Ayurveda, and my initial interest in it, flooded back. "Tell me more," I said.

Around that time, I'd been making major changes to support my mental and physical health. For years I pursued a fast-paced business career and took advantage of my body, assuming it would always show up for me when I needed it. My health had always been generally good, and I stayed on top of wellness trends that promised longevity. I identified as a "biohacker," someone who likes to experiment with how to optimize health. Then, I began experiencing more frequent respiratory illnesses and digestion issues. For treatment, I sought out holistic practitioners, which led to positive results, but I was needing something more. Martin opened a door that I hadn't known was there for me to walk through. Ayurveda was the original longevity practice, so I was intrigued to dive in with the most intensive and immersive experience there was, panchakarma.

The hospital Martin recommended was in Kerala, a southern state in India, with the best air quality in the country. It is also known to be a spiritual place. There, the cuisine, language, dress, culture, religion, and customs are different from the north, where my family is originally from, and where I have visited many times.

I had only been to Kerala once before, ten years ago, with my dad—just the two of us. My dad's family had been poor, unable to afford even domestic travel within the country, then he left India and moved to Canada when he was sixteen. So, like me, my dad had not seen much of India and had never been to the south. It was a special trip, for the two of us to bond and discover something new together. At the time, I thought I'd be back. I didn't quite know when and for what reason, until now.

Kerala is also the birthplace of Ayurveda. Between that and Martin's word, I was determined to make my way there for panchakarma. Once I got the confirmation email from the hospital, I was booked on a flight almost as quickly as I completed my sister's dare to travel to Australia.

The afternoon before I flew out of Sydney, I had a first date. Over a walk in the park, I shared with my date that I was about to go to a health retreat for a few weeks. As she asked questions, I realized I had not done much research on the place or the treatments and didn't have any details to share. She then joked that this place I was going to sounded like a scene from the television show *Nine Perfect Strangers.* It stars Nicole Kidman, playing a new-age spiritual guru, who invites nine (supposed) strangers for a retreat at her wellness center in the middle of nowhere. The staff take everyone's phones, and everyone receives extremely precise instructions for what to do. The series becomes spicy when it is revealed that Kidman's character is drugging the guests with psychedelics through their daily smoothies, which makes them hallucinate and believe they're having spiritual awakenings.

Of course, she takes it too far and crosses the line, creating exciting conflict. The guests try to escape, but fail. Kidman stays in full control of them the whole time.

My date joked that I should consider documenting my experience, "just in case you didn't make it out." As she continued to poke fun at me, I was quietly getting nervous. *What was I getting myself into?*

The next day, after my eighteen-hour flight, I decided I would, in fact, document the experience. Not out of fear for my life, but rather as a way to both remember this unique experience and share it with others. Before leaving, I'd suggested that my parents give panchakarma, or at least Ayurveda, a try. My mother's arthritis didn't seem to like the frigid Canadian winters, and the more I learned about the science, the more I wondered if her macrocosm might be affecting her microcosm. I needed evidence that it wasn't scary or dangerous. And you're currently reading that evidence.

What follows in this book are reflections on my seventeen days at the Ayurvedic hospital in India. I journaled each day I was there, not only about my treatments and daily activities, but also deeper insights into my emotions and spirituality that came through during the many hours of solitary quiet time.

After I returned home, I curated these reflections into a more coherent and concise narrative, but everything you'll read here really happened. I've only changed the names of the other patients whose stories I mention, for the sake of their privacy. I've also chosen not to share the name of this particular hospital, since it boasts a regular, long-time client base, whose ability to retreat there I don't want to interfere with. But if you'd like to know more details, I encourage you to get in touch with me directly.

Ayurveda has become more mainstream in the wellness world in the last few years, but it is not by any means well known, even amongst Indians—due to a long history of suppression of Ayurvedic practices since British colonial rule. Also, as I mentioned, the practice has its roots in the south, and so people from other regions of India may be less familiar with it.

I hope that by reading about my experience, you might learn more about Kerala, Ayurveda, panchakarma, and yoga, and perhaps be inspired to investigate your own definition of health with curiosity and sincerity. While my experience helped me gain many insights about my own imbalances, I also learned from many fellow patients, who helped me build greater compassion for others' health journeys. The more I talked with them about our experiences of living in our bodies, the more we found the kind of common ground that the whole world could benefit from.

Before I get into all the details, a few disclaimers:
I am not trained in Ayurvedic medicine or philosophy, therefore nothing I share in this book should be taken as medical advice. I simply offer my layperson's experience of panchakarma to relay my personal narrative of growth and healing. Please consult a qualified Ayurvedic practitioner if you are interested in exploring how Ayurveda and any of its treatment protocols and lifestyle or diet guidance might be helpful to you.

My experience with panchakarma was based on my unique constitution, state of health, privileges, and biases. I'm male, received the treatments in my late-thirties, and arrived with no serious medical conditions. I was the youngest person at the hospital, and every other patient had more serious health concerns than mine.

I had the financial security and freedom to be able to take time out of my life and work to come to a hospital like this as an experiment, and I went out of curiosity, rather than necessity. I could fully go offline for the few weeks required to complete the treatments thoroughly, without affecting my personal responsibilities and professional commitments. I recognize not everyone can make these choices, which will impact the accessibility of an authentic and complete panchakarma experience.

Although I'm born and raised in a Western culture, I am Indian and have visited India countless times, so I felt confident enough to navigate the entire trip. It was not a stressful experience for me, as it may be for someone who has never visited India and may not be familiar with the culture. For many, choosing to go to India for the first time for panchakarma might add layers of complication that would impede a fully healing experience. It would be wise to look closer to home for your first experience.

Day One: The Arrival
A stranger to myself

The welcome makes me feel like royalty. As the car pulls up, the door opens even before the car stops moving. Staff are lined up at the hospital entrance to receive me, all wearing smiles and dressed in white.

First, they place a garland of fresh white flowers around my neck. The smell is sweet and delicious. Then they sprinkle rose water on my head. It also smells wonderful. *The foreigners must love these hospitality niceties*, I note to myself. *Am I an Indian, or a foreigner?* I am unsure.

Ushering me inside the reception building, they ask me to exchange my shoes for bamboo slippers. Outside footwear is not allowed in the hospital—the first rule I learn.

The receptionist sits me down on a handsome but uncomfortable wicker chair. I would soon discover that this combination—nice mixed with discomfort—will become my experience for the entire stay. I sign a few waivers and liability forms. The questions pour out of me; no one answers directly, only with nods and smiles. I can't help but remember my date who made fun of me for stepping into the Indian version of *Nine Perfect Strangers*—especially when they ask me for my passport, which they keep.

Upon arriving at my room. neat and sparse, the receptionist tells me to change into my "uniform": white pajamas made of cotton and linen. He tries to sell me on the material—insisting it's very comfortable. Putting them on, I see they aren't upselling me. *Maybe I'll take a few pairs home,* I think.

Tired from a poor sleep the night before and my traveling, I fall asleep as soon as I lie down—for longer than I should have. I know this because I am woken by a doorbell. It is time for my first consultation with the doctor. Now I am groggy *and* nervous.

I know from Martin's description and my previous studies of Ayurveda that the doctors will diagnose me by looking at my face, the color of my eyes, the texture of my tongue, and the beat of my heart. Even in my half-asleep state, I know this is the worst possible moment for a doctor to diagnose me and decide my treatments for the next few weeks. But I have no choice but to flow with it.

My doctor is tall with perfectly combed and parted hair. He too is wearing white pajamas, along with a fancy white silk shawl with light embroidery around the neckline, straight out of a Bollywood movie. His demeanor while interrogating me is very warm, gentle and soft. His complexion looks radiant as well, and I couldn't stop staring at his skin. His eyes are big and bold, giving his expression a quiet confidence that complements his towering height.

The consultation lasts nearly an hour. He asks me about everything: family health history, weight, height, bowel movements, urine production, libido. He asks my blood type and is surprised I don't know. Takes my blood pressure. Measures my heart rate. After capturing these basics, he closes one of his folders, looks up at me and sighs. "Okay, now tell me why you're here."

I lean back and take a moment to respond, knowing that my response will determine, even more than these vital bodily metrics, how the next two weeks go for me.

"Immune system," I finally say. I explain to him that, in the past few years, I've experienced more frequent, more intense, and longer-lasting respiratory illnesses than ever before.

"Not a problem," he responds confidently. He starts taking notes again and explains the treatment process.

The process will involve both of us carefully listening to my body. I will have a morning consultation with him each day, where I'll describe in detail how my body feels. Then he will decide which treatments I will have for the day ahead, along with what, how much, and when I eat. He will decide what type of herbal tea or spiced water I'll drink.

That's right: I won't be drinking normal water. Despite the Kerala heat, with temperatures nearing 32 Celsius (90 Fahrenheit) daily, I'll be drinking warm ginger tea, delivered in thermal flasks twice a day to my room. Every day.

The doctor then guides me to the treatment room down the hall, where two short Indian men, who do not speak much English, greet me with hands pressed together in a prayer and guide me inside. The doctor leaves, and I am asked to fully undress before they wrap a loin cloth around my genitals. I have never worn a loin cloth before, and the image of ancient yogis comes to mind. This whole thing feels like I've time traveled.

Once I am lying face down on the massage table, the therapists start pouring warm oil on my back and arms. At first, I flinch at the heat of the oil, but I'm in no position to argue or resist. The massaging technique uses a medium pressure, unlike the deep tissue massage I am used to.

Besides the hot oil, the rubbing itself generates heat. I start to feel relaxed and calm, as one does near the end of a massage. I have no idea how much time has passed, but suddenly their hands leave my body and they're asking me to rest for five minutes to conclude the treatment. I can't really feel my body, in the best possible way—it's as if I am floating.

In a few minutes, as expected, they return to help me shower off the oil. They give me some medicated powder, which forms a paste in the water, to wash myself. They make a point to tell me not to remove *all* the oil, as the purpose is to let it soak into the skin over time.

Thank goodness for the pajamas, I think. If I had to get dressed again in my regular clothes, they would have been stained forever. I forget to use the paste on my head, so when I finally dry off and get dressed, I have a greasy Elvis-like whorl of hair. I kinda like it. I decide this will be my new look, and smile to myself.

Midday: my first meal and the first time meeting the others who are taking this Ayurvedic adventure. Another staff member coaxes me to the dining hall, which is eerily quiet.

Each person, sitting quietly in their white pajamas, has their own table and is staring out into the garden area while they eat. The only sounds I can hear are the quiet buzz of the ceiling fans and the footsteps of the staff as they bring around cups and plates.

The dining experience starts with an elegant hand-washing ritual. The server, also in white pajamas, comes over. In one hand he carries a shimmering brass jug, featuring an ornate handle and a long spout, and in the other hand a matching brass basin to catch the water. I extend my hands over the basin, and the warm water pours over my fingers. I pat my hands dry with a cloth, and I am ready to eat.

Next, the same man brings me a brass cup with warm ginger tea. I decide to make friends with this drink, as it seems we'll be spending some time together. Next comes the food, presented on a large, round steel platter. There is rice wrapped in green banana leaf, steamed green vegetables with very light seasoning, and a yellow vegetable curry. It is very pretty to look at. The serving size is small, but the taste is good, despite Martin's warnings that food might have been intentionally bland at an Ayurvedic treatment place like this.

An older Asian woman sitting on my right side asks for tea. The server comes back and says that the doctor has said she can only have tea after dinner, not after lunch. *This is serious*, I think. An innocent tea request denied. We are all instructed, as part of our protocol, to practice mindfulness while eating, which means to give full awareness to the food and not to be distracted. No speaking. No electronics. No music. No reading.

No writing. Just eating. My doctor has also told me to eat very slowly, which I used to do years ago but stopped as life got busier. I appreciated the reminder, but glacial chewing is still uncomfortable. It takes a while to finish my small meal, and I leave the dining room still a stranger to the people around me.

I go back to my room and pull out my journal, inspired to reflect for a minute about my experience so far. In the rush of booking this last-minute trip, traveling, arriving at the hospital, and being ushered around from consultation to treatment to lunch, I haven't taken a moment to ask myself, *Why am I here?*

My attempt to answer this question is threefold. First, to detox, purify, and cleanse my body. Address respiratory and digestion issues. And general preventive care for my longevity. Second, I have been curious about Ayurveda for some time, and a panchakarma is an intense immersion to satisfy this curiosity. Third, I am open to being a guinea pig to see if this type of treatment would be something that my parents might consider one day, given their age and chronic ailments. I had gently encouraged them to come with me when I started researching a trip, but, sensing their hesitation, I decided to try it first myself. I look at my reasons for being here, yet don't feel fully satisfied. I continue journaling awhile and then tears start to roll down my face as I realize the real reason I have come.

I am here to release.

Not physically, but emotionally. When I look at the other patients at the hospital in the dining hall, all of them are old and many look frail and weak. Even with my respiratory issues, I don't *need* to be here in the same way they do, but I need to be taken care of. What I truly want is space to work on my emotional health.

I've made some big professional decisions in the past few months that involved pulling the plug on several entrepreneurial projects I've invested a lot of time and money in. I had been building my identity around a lot of these projects, so pulling the plug on them means destroying parts of my identity. I feel heavy inside. Upon arriving here, I'm finally able to be alone and process what's happened. It's time to grieve for my former self.

Day Two: Liquid Gold
Swallowing the past

At 04:30 a.m., I hear loud chimes that I'm sure wakes everyone. My white pajamas are wrinkled all over: I clearly tossed and turned a lot. Surprisingly, though, I feel ready to start the day. I spend some time in my own meditation, sitting quietly on my bed, followed by some journaling and writing. Maybe one morning I'll wake up with wrinkleless white pajamas.

I stare at a fresh set of white pajamas in the corner, wrapped in tissue. Were they there yesterday, or delivered at night? Do I change into the new set now or later? I take a look in the mirror to see how disheveled I appear and decide to change after yoga, which would surely produce more wrinkles.

At 07:00 a.m., it is time for yoga. The sun is mid-rise as I walk quietly in my bamboo slippers to the yoga hall. Everyone wears their white pajamas. I try not to stare too closely to see if they are wrinkled like mine, or if they had changed into a fresh set this morning. From my quick glance around the room, it is a mix.

I've practiced yoga for years at home, but this class is completely different from the sometimes competitive and performative yoga I am used to. The teacher is a plump young Indian woman with chubby cheeks—not the thin and chiseled body type of the yoga instructors typical in New York City or LA. Another difference is that we do the practice on thin mattresses covered in bed sheets, not sticky rubber mats. The mattresses are far more comfortable. Also, there are no blocks, bolsters, or straps—which makes me nervous, until I'm assured that we don't need them because the class is so simple and gentle. Suitable for all of us, from age sixty to twenty.

Starting with neck and shoulder rolls, we move onto basic standing and seated stretches, twists, and bends. Over the course of the sixty minutes, we do something for each body part. Including *pranayama*, or intentional breathing. I am so relaxed by the end, I even doze off a bit during the final resting pose, corpse pose—where we lie on the floor like we've been prepared for burial. And if I were at home, I probably wouldn't even be out of bed yet.

After class, my appetite is on fire. The yoga poses and the warm ginger water I have been drinking must be doing their jobs. But much to my stomach's disappointment, I don't get any breakfast today. It is time to start drinking "liquid gold"—ghee, otherwise known as clarified butter—and my stomach needs to be empty.

As I sit in the treatment area waiting for the doctor, a man named Richard begins speaking with me. I don't make much eye contact, as I want to stay focused and present with my body; however, he is clearly eager to engage with me, so I turn and respond with a kind smile.

I learn that Richard has been living in Hong Kong for forty-nine years, though his accent sounds American. More interestingly, this is his sixth time here at the hospital. He looks in pretty good shape. *A good sign, I think, especially if my parents come one day.* I ask him why he keeps coming back.

He says, "Everyone says I look amazing after I do one of these. My eyes glow. My skin shines. My hair is beautiful." He is a walking endorsement for the hospital, and for Ayurveda.

Then he gets down to business and warns me in a whisper, "The ghee you're about to drink is the most disgusting thing you'll ever have in your life. When they give you the cardamom and lime to chase it, take extra."

Before I have time to clarify what he means, the doctor arrives for the morning consultation. He takes out his notebook and, without making eye contact, starts questioning me with long pauses in between.

"Sleep?" is the first one.

"Fine, normal, eight hours," I respond. I watch him write the number 8 in his notebook.

"Appetite?"

"Normal, I think." Right now, I've never been hungrier in my life. Is this "normal"?

"Bowels?"

I paused. "Normal." He writes it down.

"Stick out your tongue," he orders. I do and his serious face doesn't change. A good sign, I hope.

"Okay, time to drink the ghee."

My heart picks up its pace—I am nervous about what's coming, thanks to Richard.

I am taken to a new treatment room, this one with a large wooden table in the middle of the room. The middle is slightly hollowed out into the perfect shape for a body. I wonder which day I'll have a treatment on this inviting piece of wood.

With a beaker of warm ghee in his hand, the doctor asks me to sit on a stool. The thin layer of golden liquid is far less intimidating than I expected. Standing in front of me, he closes his eyes and chants a prayer. I close my eyes too. I think we are praying for different things.

He hands me the drink. I stare at it for a second and then bring the beaker to my mouth, take a deep breath, and swallow a giant gulp of the stuff. I can't take it all in one shot, it is too much, so I take it in two gulps. I do it quickly.

And then, relief. There's barely any aftertaste. "I've had food that tastes far worse than that," I say to the doctor.

The doctor smiles—another relief. "Yes, I know. Everyone makes a big deal out of the taste, but it's not a big deal at all."

I wash it down with some warm water. He doesn't offer the cardamom lime chaser, and I don't ask for it. I am fine.

The doctor tells me repeatedly not to sleep for the next two hours, despite any fatigue, as that will lower my body temperature. Which could be bad. Ghee, after all, is clarified *butter*. A memory from childhood comes to mind. We always had a metal bowl of ghee in the kitchen cabinet beside the spices. And the ghee was always in solid form, never liquid. Room temperature ghee solidifies—something I don't want to happen inside my body.

When it's time to walk, I go readily to keep my body warm. My mission is to not let the ghee solidify inside my digestive tract.

A few hours later, my body has worked through the ghee and is hungry again, just in time for lunch. After I am done with the meal, I am invited to meet the chef for a food consultation. We sit at a table inside, across from each other, and he explains some of the Ayurvedic principles used in the kitchen. He tells me food is medicine—that is the philosophy. Food is not meant to taste good. It's not meant to taste bad, either, but one doesn't eat for pleasure. One eats for healing.

All the meals served at the hospital are vegetarian, mostly vegan. They use only fresh produce, either grown in the hospital grounds or bought from local growers. The food is only prepared one hour before mealtime to ensure maximum freshness and benefits.

Each person's meals are personalized and decided by their doctor after the daily consultation. No changes are allowed, though we are allowed to ask for seconds, or even thirds to satisfy our appetites. I make a mental note to remember this for the next meal, as I am already starting to feel hungry. Any issues with the food choices, he says, you must take it up with your doctor at the following consultation. Not even the chef has any leeway to experiment or express his own creativity through the food.

He says that eating food by hand, versus using utensils, supports the goal of healing. Touching food with the fingers sends a signal to the brain that food is coming soon, which generates saliva in the mouth, which in turn aids digestion. So much of Ayurveda is about digestion, I'm learning.

I've been eating Indian food my entire life but have generally leaned towards using utensils more than my hands, like all Westerners. However, after this tidbit of information, I'm motivated to use my hands more.

Next, I have a consultation with the yoga teacher.

This one is briefer. I share with her that I have been practicing yoga for ten years, did my yoga teacher training five years ago, have been practicing meditation daily for ten years, and now teach meditation. I even have a book on meditation in the works.

She smiles, happy to hear about my enthusiasm and experience. "You'll find all of the practices very gentle and simple," she says and explains that the purpose of yoga here is to support the treatments. It's not a stand-alone activity to get exercise; it is all in support of the detox and cleanse.

I take another lap around the hospital to make sure the lunch and ghee are all cooking well inside my body. But almost immediately upon returning to my room and sitting at my desk, I'm awash with fatigue. They warned me that the ghee would make me tired. It seemed like a harmless warning initially, but what is happening inside my body does not feel harmless.

Because it is so dense, ghee requires a disproportionate amount of energy to digest in the stomach. The process deprives the rest of the body of blood flow and energy. The effects of the ghee then spread to the rest of the body, acting as a detoxifying lubricant, and it binds to the toxins everywhere. They are then purged through the liver, kidney, skin, and bowels.

That's why we're told to not do any excessive physical activity or tire out the body. The doctor explained to me that's why there's no gym or swimming pool in the hospital. And it explains why the yoga is very gentle. They go as far as to advise avoiding unnecessary talking and thinking during the ghee days, hence the encouragement to disconnect from devices, to not listen to music, to not read too much, and so on. All these activities consume energy that the body desperately needs to process and detoxify with the ghee. In order to digest fully, we need to rest. If it sounds intense, it is because it is.

A few hours later, that ghee doesn't feel so pure and innocent.

During my afternoon oil massage, I start to connect some dots. The ghee is pulling toxins from the body internally, and with the massage, the oil pulls out toxins through the body's largest organ: the skin. Same process, different entry point.

After the massage, I feel deeply relaxed. They cover me in a white sheet for the rest period. I can't help but laugh to myself, as I doze in and out of sleep, thinking about how it's ironic that attempting to improve my life involves so much lying around like a corpse.

Day Three: The Palace
Giving myself fully

While waiting for my morning dose of ghee today, I meet an elderly Indian woman who speaks with a British accent. She's been receiving panchakarma for twenty years now. When I ask her why she keeps coming back, she gives me a surprising answer: "I don't know any different." She doesn't know what the benefits are because she hasn't experienced life without regular panchakarma detox. As she can tell I am not satisfied with her first response, she adds, "Coming here allows me to feel more connected within myself. I come feeling disjointed and in multiple pieces. I leave feeling like a single piece."

Now that's an endorsement.

I want to keep talking with this woman, but my doctor walks into the waiting room, ready to see me.

We debrief on the status of my bowels, urine, digestion, and energy. I do not feel shy about sharing these details anymore. "I'm ready to increase the intensity of the treatments. This feels too easy," I say to the doctor. "I'm healthy and young and have the mental and physical capacity to handle more."

He doesn't acknowledge my bravery.

Yesterday, I received 25 mL of ghee. Today, he gives me 60 mL. I think that was 10 mL more than he had originally planned, thanks to the confidence I showed in being able to handle more. As he gives me the beaker to drink, I joke, "So tomorrow, we do 100 mL." He laughs out loud and says, "You're in a hurry," then turns away without letting me respond. We'll see if my negotiation attempt works tomorrow.

As I leave the treatment building to begin my prescribed walking rounds—I must complete ten rounds today, since there's much more ghee to move—one of the staff stops me and asks to give me a tour of the campus. *Perfect timing.*

"Can I have my running shoes?" I ask her, remembering that they took them yesterday and I had not seen them since. I imagine I'll be more comfortable walking in them than my slippers. She nods, and we head to the reception desk.

After retrieving my shoes, I work up the courage to ask for my passport back. I'm not sure if keeping it is intentional or accidental, so I speak in my firm, non-

nonsense business voice, not wanting to give them the option to say no to me. "I think you forgot to give me back my passport yesterday," I say. She knows exactly where my passport is and returns with it. *What a relief.*

Running shoes secured, I followed the woman on a walk around the campus, a former palace, and learn about its history. In the fifteenth century, two centuries before the British invaded India, the original palace was constructed by a king from a different part of Kerala. He was an officer in some other government and had a disease. Back then, if someone had a disease, they were deemed unfit to govern, so he was told to leave his post.

With the aim of curing his disease, he traveled all over the state and was told to come to this area because of its healing properties. He spent four days in the forest, where many medicinal trees naturally grow, and supposedly emerged cured of his disease. He fell in love with the area, convinced of its healing energy.

Once he was well, he returned to government work and lobbied to be in charge of developing this area he discovered. Over the next several centuries, the palace—now the main building of the panchakarma center—stayed in his family, sustained by the profits from abundant tea plantations. However, once the British showed up in the eighteenth century, the palace got into financial trouble and the family had to sell off different buildings; the once-royal family eventually lived in the palace grounds. The newer, whiter, taller colonial buildings built for the British still stand on the land today.

Fast-forward to the late-nineteenth century. The then-king passed away, and his son, his heir, was only thirteen years old. A minor was not allowed to take the throne, so the boy's older sister was made queen.

Until then, patriarchal culture was extremely strong in most of India. Women were not allowed to speak in the presence of men, had to study and eat in separate rooms, and were not allowed to make eye contact with men. They were treated as a lower social class.

Once the deceased king's daughter was made queen, the culture shifted to a matriarchy, with women in charge. For example, in traditional Indian culture, especially back then, daughters were married off and sent to their new husband's home to live with her in-laws and give them grandchildren. After the regime change, when the daughters in the extended family were married, their new husbands moved into the palace.

Many signs of matriarchy remain around the hospital grounds. For example, there is an area for music—a hobby for the women—that is located in the main part of the palace, right in the center.

As the palace was broken up into smaller and smaller pieces, many hoteliers started eyeing the property. In the 1990s, they continued to make offers to the family to buy the entire plot. However, the original family that owned the palace was Brahmin, the highest class in Indian culture and one that doesn't tolerate the consumption of meat, alcohol, tobacco, or the use of leather products, so they said no to every single offer from a hotel.

Then in 2000, a businessman in Kerala discovered the palace, having heard—like the first king—that the location had healing properties. He offered to build an Ayurvedic hospital on the grounds, which was accepted by the family. They gave him a sixty-year lease. It took four years to reconstruct and rehabilitate the buildings and grounds, and the hospital has been operating for twenty years now. The group has four Ayurvedic hospitals in total in the South of India.

There are over 100 staff for the 19 guest rooms and a maximum of 24 patients at any time. That's a decent staff-patient ratio, four to one, and you can feel it in the care and attentiveness of everyone's service—from the treatments to the cooking to the neatly folded pajamas.

During the tour, I also see the hospital's extensive water filtration system, which uses a complex combination of charcoal, sand, and bamboo. I also see how the Ayurvedic medicines used in the treatments are made, including the oils. There is a hut with giant cauldrons full of hot oil, boiling over a wood fire. Oils take seven to nine days to make, with multiple steps of preparation, purification, and infusion with medicinal ingredients.

After the tour, I feel more connected to my temporary home.

It has now been forty-eight hours since I arrived at the hospital. I have been wearing the same white pajamas, and I have not engaged with the digital world the whole time. No phone, no email, no WhatsApp, no social media, no media at all. There is no way for anyone in my world to reach me, and no way for me to be distracted by the digital noise that I have become accustomed to hearing.

To disconnect for seventeen days took preparation. I only had about a week between booking my trip and leaving, so I hurried to put pieces in place with the teams in my respective businesses—the lawyers, the bankers, the real estate agents, and more. I also gave my parents, sister, and close friends a heads up that I'd be fully offline during this time. A few cousins in Delhi were sent the details of the retreat center, and a message from me saying I'll be listing them as my emergency contacts. There were over 100 people I felt I had to notify in advance of going off grid.

I did not have to take such extreme measures, but I believe that I have to be fully present with the experience and my emotions for this Ayurvedic experiment to work. I want to treat it not only as a physical cleanse but also, equally important, a mental and emotional cleanse. So, I am all in.

Taking things a step further, I have disconnected from my self-prescribed health routines. Over the past year, I've built a team of doctors, nutritionists, herbalists, and specialists to support my inconsistent immune system and optimize my health, following mainstream wellness trends. Along the way, I've built my own pharmacy of supplements that I take everywhere: twenty-five to thirty pills a day. I am curious to see what happens to my body without them.

I even took off my sleep and fitness tracker, a ring that I've been wearing continuously for two years. Although there's a geeky part of me that is curious to see my heart rate, sleep score, activity score, breathing, and other metrics during this treatment, there's a nurturing part of me that knows I'll feel more at ease mentally if I'm not being tracked.

I'm giving myself fully to this experience. A sign that I'm not attached to any routines, be it checking email, responding to WhatsApp messages, popping pills, or analyzing my sleep data. To be attached to these external metrics isn't being healthy, even if it is in the name of wellness.

Day Four: Panchakarma
Everything must go

My journey with yoga started ten years ago. My girlfriend at the time was a long-time yogi, but I was not open to it at all. I would go to classes with her kicking and screaming, claiming I was only doing her a favor. As fate would have it, shortly after that relationship ended, I discovered my own passion for yoga and began a regular practice.

I was living in Toronto and found a studio between my apartment and my office; I started taking class every other morning. I would travel often to New York and London and found yoga studios there as well. I began to go on yoga retreats, immersing myself into more intensive practice environments. My nightly reading began to include yoga philosophy, which is how I discovered that yoga is a set of principles of how to live. Physical postures are only one of the eight branches or "limbs" of yoga, which include *yamas* (a set of social ethics), *niyamas* (a set of personal practices), *asana* (postures), *samadhi* (harmony), *dhyana* (letting go), *dharana* (concentration), *prathyahara* (turning inward), and *pranayama*, which works with your energy and mind through the breath. Here at the hospital, there are the morning *asana* practices and forty-five-minute pranayama practices every afternoon at 5:00 p.m. They exercises are gentle, guided, and effortless for me. Afterwards I feel alive, centered, and balanced. Only a few days in, and I'm inspired to reincorporate daily and pranayama practices when I leave this place. I have lost touch with this discipline over the past few years as life got busier, and I am reminded now of why I love them so much: they help me feel grounded and calm, and taking the time each morning to do them feels like I'm setting myself up to succeed in every way.

Today after class, everyone is in a chatty mood, so I make some more friends.

First is Nathan—a tall, confident man with white stubble on his pale face. He wears prayer beads around his neck, and his presence is gentle but firm. He is French but has been in New York for thirty-five years and now splits his time between Athens and New York.

His wife is Greek, and she is also here for treatment. They came last year for the first time and had such a positive experience that they booked this visit the day after they left.

His first panchakarma happened after he'd retired from thirty-five years of working in a large public corporation, most recently as CEO of two divisions. While we don't connect much on professional topics, we do connect on spiritual ones. Here we were, two CEOs walking around in our white pajamas at an Ayurvedic hospital in the south of India, not talking business but talking energy.

He shares with me about Amma, the "hugging saint," who is based in Kerala. I have heard about her in passing over the years but never looked into her story. Coincidentally, or perhaps not, a few days before coming to Kerala, my Canadian friend was telling me about Amma and encouraged me to go give her a hug. Nathan spent five days at Amma's ashram before coming to the hospital. He has lots to say about the entire campus, which houses thousands of people in Amma's village, and all of the inspiring work she's done in building schools and hospitals. He was so touched by his experience there that he has decided to cut his hospital visit short by two days so he can take his wife to see Amma for the first time after they are done here. He invites me to join them, and I say yes.

My one-word theme for this year is "flow," and this feels like the perfect flow decision. I had intentionally not made any plans after the hospital, and now I know why.

Time for more ghee.

During the morning consultation, I tell the doctor about a concern I have: "I'm always hungry. I had four rotis last night, asked for extra rice porridge for lunch, and I still don't feel full." I've never had such a strong appetite before and wonder if something isn't working the way it should.

"Good," he responds blankly. "We are trying to increase your digestive fire."

"What do you mean?"

"Your ghee has been medicated with herbs that stimulate hunger. And the ginger water you've been drinking for three days also stimulates your digestive system."

Then I guess it's working very well, I think.

He then reminds me that it's better to not discuss treatments and symptoms with other patients. For example, for a patient who may be here to lose weight, their ghee will be medicated with herbs that suppress their appetite. This really is personalized medicine, even without the fancy diagnostic testing I am used to. In my morning walk with Nathan, we discussed how talking about our personal treatment experiences isn't helpful. It can easily cause anxiety and worry for people, especially those new to it. I've noticed a few of the other patients are often complaining about their symptoms and interviewing others to compare. Basically, the opposite of what the doctors advise.

Yesterday, I had 60 mL of ghee. I try to negotiate for a larger dose today, to intensify the effects. "Let's do 120 mL today, doctor," I say while his back is turned to me.

"Ha, you'll vomit if you take that much today," he says. Without thinking, I respond, "I'm fine to vomit, a little at least." And then realize how gross that sounds. I would take it back if I could.

In what seems like a compromise, I receive 90 mL of ghee. Again, it goes down fine in three big gulps. I intentionally wait an extra few seconds before washing it down with warm water, to prove I don't mind the taste in the hope that he'll up the dosage tomorrow.

Later that evening, a doctor gives a talk to explain more to the patients about panchakarma. The ghee treatment, it turns out, is only preparation for the real detox. I had done no research in advance about the actual treatments, but I remember a conversation I had when booking the treatment. They'd wanted me to stay for eighteen days, which I thought was too long to be away from work. I countered with fourteen but then agreed to seventeen in order to do the preparation they said was necessary. Now I understand their insistence; if I'd only had one day of ghee, my purgation might not be completed.

Now it is time to learn what I actually signed up for.

The word panchakarma is Sanskrit: *pancha* means "five" and *karma* denotes "action or procedure." It translates to "five actions" or "five treatments."

This purification process is a core therapy in Ayurveda, eliminating toxins from the body by balancing the three *doshas* (*vata*, *pitta*, and *kapha*). Ayurvedic texts that detail these procedures and their many variations emphasize their significance in maintaining and restoring physical, mental, and emotional balance when used properly. Ayurveda maintains that true healing is only possible when we address the root cause of imbalance, not just the symptoms. Western medicine, as many of my doctor friends complain to me often about, is really about symptom management. Ayurveda is different—maybe that's why I've been so drawn to it.

The essence of panchakarma, as with all Ayurveda, is in its personalized approach. It's not a one-size-fits-all protocol, but rather a tailored set of therapies, aligned with an individual's unique constitution, imbalances, and specific health concerns. I love how this philosophy of health acknowledges the uniqueness of each person.

These are the five panchakarma treatments:

1. Vamana (Therapeutic Vomiting)

Vamana is a controlled process that eliminates excess mucus. It's particularly helpful for issues like congestion, asthma, or certain skin diseases. Imagine the body as a garden at the end of winter; vamana is like removing a stagnant layer of damp weeds and dead leaves, allowing the garden to breathe and flourish. The process involves loosening and mobilizing the toxins, followed by drinking a therapeutic concoction. This triggers vomiting, clearing out mucus and toxins from the respiratory and gastrointestinal tracts.

2. Virechana (Purgation Therapy)

Virechana is the gentle cleansing of the lower digestive tract. It's especially good for imbalances, like liver disorders or skin conditions. Think of it as a deep cleanse for the digestive system, flushing out toxins and excess bile through the bowels. After preparing the body, the patient consumes a strong natural laxative, and they have many bowel movements until they're empty. It's a reset button for digestion, helping the body to absorb nutrients and feel more energetic.

3. Basti (Medicated Enema)

Basti involves administering herbal decoctions and oils through the rectum. It nourishes and hydrates the colon, which is believed to be the root of health in Ayurveda. This treatment addresses issues like joint disorders, constipation, and neurological ailments. It's like irrigating a field, ensuring that every plant gets the nourishment it needs to grow strong and healthy.

4. Nasya (Nasal Administration)

Nasya involves the introduction of medicated oils, decoctions, or powders into the nostrils. It's particularly good for issues above the neck, such as sinus blockage, headaches, or even brain fog. The nose is a direct route to the brain and consciousness, so the medicines have a strong effect. The medicated substance is gently administered into the nostrils, penetrating the sinus, throat, and head regions. This not only cleanses the pathways but also nourishes the tissues, bringing clarity and lightness. *Nasya* can also be done daily, in a gentler way, at home.

5. Rakta Mokshana (Bloodletting)

Rakta mokshana is the process of purification used for conditions where toxins are believed to have accumulated in the blood. This can be done in a controlled and safe environment using techniques like leech therapy, which is rare these days. It's considered effective for certain skin conditions, hypertension, and other blood-related disorders.

As the doctor describes the options, I'm eager to try them all and get the full detox effect, but am disappointed to learn that not everyone does all of the treatments. I'm curious about which ones I'll be doing.

I've tried asking the doctor every day so far, to which he always responds with some version of "we'll see based on how your body feels and is reacting."

Day Five: Heart to Heart
A pulse outside myself

I'm starting to feel the ghee.

This morning is the first time I do not feel well when I wake up. Sleep was disturbed. My appetite is significantly lower, my body more fatigued. My body is directing energy and blood flow to my stomach to digest the increasing amounts of ghee, and this reduces blood flow to the brain. The doctor kept asking me the past few days if I was having headaches, and now I know why.

Today I receive 120 mL of ghee. I take it like a champ, without so much as a grimace. But I make no attempt to negotiate for more.

I make my morning walking rounds extra slowly, as my whole aching body feels stiff, and think about how nice it is to not have to change clothes and look presentable while undergoing this process. White pajamas every day, all day—I've come to love them! I never had a school uniform growing up, never worked a job that had a dress code. I always imagined this to be a way of enforcing conformity, but all I feel in my white pajamas is a sense of *freedom*.

Also, I'm also now fine with my hair being oily and my skin a little smelly. We're all walking a ton in the sun and sometimes not allowed to shower after massage oil treatments. I wonder how the world would be if we all accepted our bodies like this, in their natural states.

While walking, I also reflect that to be a good patient here at the hospital, I need to learn to *be* patient. The connection between the two meanings of the word "patient" had never hit me until this moment. I've been very fortunate and never actually been an inpatient at a hospital; the rare times I've been to a hospital have been either been as an outpatient for minor procedures or to visit someone else. And while I'm not sick or injured now, my health is dependent on the doctors and other staff here. I'm not in charge of my life right now; it's in their hands, and trusting their decisions has created some friction in me. I'm not used to being vulnerable.

I'm rarely patient in my daily life. From the moment I wake up to the moment I go to sleep, urgency drives me. Whatever routine activity I do throughout the day,

I often carry out all of them with a frenetic energy. Here, that doesn't fly. Even if there were something to be urgent about (there's no penalty for showing up late to yoga, meals, or treatments, urgency and stress would negate the treatments I've come for. I'm not here to take care of things; I'm here to be taken care of.

When I look back to my first journal entry, I see that I was looking forward to being taken care of fully: not being responsible for my food, activities, treatments, and decisions. But it's been more of an adjustment to release control and give myself fully over to the hospital staff than I thought. I am slowly learning to be more a *patient* patient.

There is a Hindu temple in the hospital grounds, and a priest is there each morning and afternoon for about one hour. An older Indian man with long white hair, he sits cross-legged near the altar in his loose white pants.

The first few days, I simply passed by and stared at the temple—and the priest inside. But today on my walk, I step inside. I tiptoe inside the temple gate, take off my bamboo slippers, and walk up the stairs quietly.

The priest greets me with a gentle smile and nod, a silent invitation to come up to the altar. First, I study the altar. It's adorned with fresh white flowers and several lit candles. Red and gold decorations cover the inside wall. And watching over it all is a statue of Kali, the fierce goddess of destruction. The destruction of evil, that is.

I bring my palms together, close my eyes, bow my head, and begin to pray.

The posture brings back memories of childhood. I was raised Hindu, and our home has had a temple for as long as I can remember. When I was eight years old, my grandmother set up an altar for me in my bedroom while she was visiting. I prayed each morning before going to school for ten years.

We always visited the community Hindu temple every few weeks as a family. My uncle had been the architect of the Hindu temple in Ottawa, and our families were active in the local Indian community. Each Sunday, a different family would host the lunch service, which meant cooking for 300 to 400 people. I have so many childhood memories of the temple, particularly the few weekends per year when we would host. The quantity of food my parents cooked was insane. My sister and I would both be given jobs to do, such as setting up the plates and napkins. As we got older, we would serve the rice, and as we got even older, we would serve one of the curries. Watching my parents effortlessly host a lunch for hundreds of people made it feel normal to me growing up.

Now, standing with my eyes closed and hands connected in a prayer pose, I remember all those childhood experiences and appreciate how the temple connected me to my family, culture, and religion.

My prayers today start with gratitude for my health and the chance to have this experience. Then for the staff and people involved to make the hospital run. Then, fitting to the goddess Kali, I began to pray for the destruction of any harm that might come my way, and then my family's way and then in the way of the other patients here. As my prayers expand beyond me, I notice a shift in my energy. The fatigue from the day has gone, and I now feel light and energized. My hands are on my heart, supported by the inclusion of others' hands and hearts.

That's the power of prayer: shifting the energy within yourself and in the world around you. In this way, prayer becomes a form of giving.

After dinner, there is to be a classical Indian music performance, which I am looking forward to.

South Indian classical music, referred to as Carnatic music, is a sophisticated art form that I find interesting. My friend, Raghu, whom I've known since I was four years old, is a Carnatic music singer. Through him over the years, I've been exposed to this form of vocal-centric music, which is considered one of the world's oldest and most developed musical systems.

Carnatic music can be traced back to ancient Vedic Indian texts and is based on the system of *ragas*, a melodic frameworks that provide musicians with a set of rules for building a tune. Each *raga* is said to evoke specific feelings and emotions. The rhythm in Carnatic music is governed by the *tala* system. A tala is a cyclical rhythmic pattern that consists of beats (or counts) that are grouped in specific ways to create different rhythmic cycles. Raga plus tala equals melody plus rhythm—a song.

A significant portion of a Carnatic music performance is the presentation of *kritis*, or compositions. However, improvisation plays a crucial role, with artists skillfully showcasing their creativity within the framework of the raga and tala. I love improv, and this is what makes Carnatic music really interesting to listen to, if you know what you're looking for. The lead vocal singer is improvising each composition, and the others who are accompanying him or her have to repeat the composition back to the lead singer using their instruments. It's like a free-form conversation between the artists.

Listening to the music tonight feels like another kind of prayer—a submission into a flow bigger than me, bigger than all of us here.

As I walk back to my room after the performance, I befriend a tall German man named Patrick and his wife, Sophia. I had noticed them the past few days, sitting on one side of the dining hall in their white pajamas, at the same spot for every meal, with serious faces. I had judged them as grumpy and not happy to be here. I could not have been more wrong. It is their fifth visit to the hospital, and they've been here already for twenty-eight days. That's the longest duration of any of the other patients I have met so far. As we talk and get to know each other, Patrick laughs and smiles, congenially hitting my shoulder often. His persona is completely different from what I had assumed. A reminder to not judge a book by its cover. At one point, he leans toward me and whispers, "I only speak with the people I like and feel have really good energy."

I smile, as I sense there is a compliment in there. Being Canadian, I come from a culture that's known as friendly and warm. Combine that with my curious personality, and I easily make friends with most everyone I meet. However, I'm not here to make friends and haven't been going out of my way to be social. But I understand what Patrick means about being intentional about the energy I surround myself with. I'm grateful he planted the seed into my awareness early in the visit. He also feels inspired to share some of his life wisdom with me. In me, he says he sees a ready listener. I am genuinely curious what is going to come out of this tall serious German man's mouth next.

"It doesn't matter how much money you have, or who you are, but rather *how* you are . . . in the heart." He places his hand over his heart and beams a warm smile at me.

I needed this dose of liquid gold.

Day Six: The Pond
Reflections not my own

The effects of the ghee are strengthening now. Headaches. Muscle stiffness and soreness all over. Loss of appetite. Loose bowels. Sensitive stomach. Lack of mental focus and clarity. Nausea.

I think for sure that with all these changes, I would be done with the ghee treatments and ready for the real panchakarma. I am wrong. When I share my condition with my doctor in the morning consultation, his reply surprises me: "Okay, one more day of ghee and then we're done."

I sigh and give myself a little pep talk as I drag myself to the treatment room for the now all-too-familiar routine.

"How much today?" I ask with a note of annoyance in my voice.

"Only a bit more than yesterday, 140 mL," the doctor responds, not looking my way to see my facial expression.

I do a quick mental calculation:

140 mL on day 6 + 120 mL on day 5 + 90 mL on day 4 + 60 mL on day 3 + 25 mL on day 2 + = 435 mL.

That's nearly half a liter of medicated, clarified butter! And to think that after the first and second days, I was trying to negotiate for more. Now I am trying to negotiate for less. All of this is so new to me, including being unsuccessful in negotiations.

I drink the ghee and prepare for the worst. But, surprisingly, today the symptoms are not as rough as the previous day. I feel fine—I mean, not normal by any means, but glad that we did another day of ghee to try and maximize the detoxification benefits.

As I start to do my walking rounds, in my white pajamas as always, I bump into one of the staff members. She is friendly and in a talkative mood, and she unapologetically joins me for my walk.

Despite feeling bloated and nauseated, I focus on being a listener in this conversation, for I fear that I speak, something other than words might come out of my mouth. I ask her where she's from. It's not Kerala, but another state in southern India. My sense of the geography of India is quite poor, mostly because both my parents are from Delhi, my extended family is in Delhi, and nearly all of my twenty or so visits to India have been only to Delhi. I've hardly set foot in the south.

She shares that she got married two years ago. Time for the juicy question I know will get her really talking: "How did you meet your husband?" I smile in anticipation of the story.

"Arranged marriage," she says, in a serious matter-of-fact way. My smile fell.

My curiosity is piqued. "Like, how arranged? Arranged-arranged? Or, like, introduced?"

"Arranged-arranged."

"Tell me more. You know, I've only seen arranged marriages in the movies. Despite being Indian, I don't think I know anyone who has had a fully arranged marriage. What was the process like?"

She sighs, then gives me a crash course in arranged marriages. As I listen, I feel like we've stepped back in time 100 years. But no, this was a mere two years ago. It is mind-blowing to hear.

Her sister had found the match on an online matrimonial site. They're not called "dating apps" in India, as the concept of dating is not widely accepted, at least not in the more traditional regions. A matrimonial website is what it sounds like—a place to find a husband or wife. The other major difference is that she was not using it; her family were using it for her. Likewise the man she married.

The match identified by her sister looked interesting in terms of personality, prospects, and appearance. That was step one. Step two: her parents spoke with his parents over the phone. Step three: the meeting.

The boy, with an entourage of around fifteen people, including parents, uncles, aunts, and cousins showed up at her parents' home. Waiting for them was her entourage, of similar size and composition.

"I was so nervous. When they all showed up, I didn't even know which one was the boy meant for me; my uncle had to point him out to me from the window."

Everyone exchanged pleasantries, and then the girl and the boy had a chance to speak in private. Well, semi-private. For ten whole minutes. She had ten minutes to say yes or no.

"What did you talk about?" I ask enthusiastically.

"I made my demands very clear. I explained that my sister is married to someone in the army, and if something were to happen, then he would have to also take care of her. And that I would want him to treat my family as his. If he said yes to those two demands, then I would say yes."

He said yes. She said yes. Deal done.

"That sounds like a business transaction!" I blurt out. She doesn't react. Only afterwards do I realize why—it was a business transaction, and she knows it.

A few months later, the formal engagement happened. The two of them were not allowed to speak or meet between that initial ten-minute business meeting and the engagement ceremony. In that period, the parents met a few times, including a visit to his parents' home to see how they lived because she'd be moving in with her in-laws.

"You must have been able to speak with each other at the engagement," I say.

"Not really. There were a lot of family members there, so we were each busy with our respective relatives."

In her culture's tradition, the marriage happens within forty days of the engagement. So, within two months of their first ten-minute chat, they were married. I think back to the many business deals I've done in my career—none closed so quickly.

She then moved in with her husband and her in-laws. Her sister joined her for the first week, to help with the "adjustment," to put it mildly. She was twenty-seven at the time and had never lived outside of her parents' home.

As I thank her for sharing her story with me and walk back to my room alone, I realize how grateful I am to have been born and raised in Canada. My parents migrated from Delhi to Montreal one month before I was born. Each time I visited India growing up, I imagined what my life might have looked like had my parents stayed. Now my curiosity about arranged marriages has been satisfied, leaving nothing left to wonder about on this topic. Ever.

In the afternoon, I join a karma yoga session. Karma yoga isn't at all about physical movement; it's a branch of yoga that is dedicated to serving others—the yoga of giving with no expectation of getting anything in return. This is where our common notion of karma comes from—"what goes around comes around" and "you reap what you sow." In the original context, the focus of karma yoga is on giving positive energy, without the expectation of receiving it back in this life, to create more positive conditions for future embodiments of one's soul.

The karma yoga practice is at 4:30 p.m. every afternoon by the pond. I'm excited that today I'm not too tired from treatments to go check it out. The pond is large, although the water level is quite low—a good twenty feet below where we stand alongside the edge. We feed the fish and ducks with rice.

The act of grabbing some rice and throwing it into the pond has more gravity to it than I imagined. The physical act of direct giving is very different from a more removed act of, say, an online donation, and it inspires something within me. I start to feel emotional. I start to feel more connected to everyone around me. And most of all, I feel inspired to give more once I get back home.

Day Seven: Identity
A name left behind

Between 08:00 and 09:00 a.m. is peak social hour. After yoga and breakfast, everyone is desperate for some live connection, given the dining hall is a talk-free zone. Before our respective treatments start, the morning hour is the only time that everyone is free to walk and talk without the risk of feeling too oily, bloated, or tired to engage.

As most of the other patients are from Europe, it also makes sense they are more social at this hour given the time difference; their loved ones at home are still sleeping, so they have no one else to talk to. The temperature is also pleasant and inviting enough for a walk before the sun gets too hot.

The short trip from my room to the dining hall for breakfast takes me more than thirty minutes because I stop to greet at least a half-dozen fellow patients, all dressed in white pajamas, all eager to chit-chat. I can see who's showered and changed that morning, as their white pajamas are nicely pressed and wrinkle-free. And the rest of us, me included, wear white pajamas that are full of wrinkles from sleeping. But it's a no-judgment zone, so everyone smiles all the same.

Today is my first day without ghee. Hoorah! Today is also my first time having breakfast since I arrived. It's a bowl of steamed apples, a generous serving, and I wonder how I will feel eating this after all the ghee of the past five days. The breakfast is quite soothing. The apples are warm, easy to digest, and not too sweet.

After the morning consultation with the doctor, I have my first of two massages for the day—both four-handed massages. I do the math. Two people, massaging me simultaneously, on two separate occasions, for one hour each, is the equivalent of a four-hour massage. It's heavenly, except for one issue: the purpose of the massages is no longer relaxation, like the first few I had upon arriving; now the aim is detoxification. This means that the pressure and force they use is very strong, as if trying to squeeze toxins directly out of my skin.

It isn't painful, but it isn't comfortable either. I note, based on the smell, that a different oil is used in the morning and afternoon sessions.

Between massages I meet Sheila, a Californian who has been living in Paris for forty-two years. Nevertheless, she still speaks at double speed, like an American, and her eyes dart from left to right constantly. I wonder why she's here, since she looks healthy and fit, physically—but so do I. When I ask her, she says it is for her mental health. She doesn't appear down or depressed, but rather up. Maybe too up, actually.

As we get to talking, I share that I have disconnected completely from my phone and my world since I arrived almost a week ago. When she describes how connected she is on a normal basis, I can see why she is here. I gently nudge her to consider disconnecting from her devices.

She pauses for the first time in our conversation, and says, "You know what? You've inspired me. I'm going to disconnect, not fully, but a lot more than I would have otherwise had I not met you. Thank you." She then continues to talk, this time about the boiled apples she had for breakfast this morning. I have never seen someone so excited about boiled apples before.

At lunch, I notice that the older people always sit at the exact same spot in the dining hall. I guess the elderly don't like change very much and get set in their ways. I wonder if I'll be like that one day.

Today in particular everyone looks frail and weak sitting in their white pajamas. It isn't just their age, I realize. Many of us are finishing our ghee, and a few have had their purgation day. Although each person's treatment is customized, these preparatory phases follow a similar cadence, hence why we're all in sync. This midway point of the protocol is apparently the lowest point, and it's obvious: people's faces are droopy, they walk slowly—myself included—and everyone generally looks devoid of energy. I know my low point is coming soon.

Looking around at everyone's drawn faces, all of us at our own tables, dressed in our white pajamas, eating slowly in silence, without any phones, any conversation, any music, any books—I suddenly feel a total loss of inspiration.

It feels like we are all being punished. Not for crimes but for how we've taken advantage of and ignored our bodies. That's karma. We are here to heal, strengthen, and purify our bodies and minds—and we were the root causes of our own suffering.

Healing the root cause means taking away our independence, at least for a while. We're all walking the grounds in our white pajamas, not allowed to choose our clothes or leave. The only human contact we have is with the staff and with the other patients occasionally. We get morsels of food, at predefined hours. What we eat is not of our own choosing but of the doctors'. Any attempt to negotiate for different food is refused. We're told to not speak most of the time and to be only with ourselves. We're encouraged to not work and cannot have devices in any of the public spaces. We are ushered from treatment to treatment, none of which are particularly pleasant—mildly painful and uncomfortable.

And the irony is that we all admitted ourselves to this place. We came of our own volition. My previous motivation dimmed; I wonder in desperation, What's going on here? That question itself, I think, is part of our healing.

As I continue to sit in silence, quietly eating my meal and staring at all these old people, I began to wonder about identity. We hold on to our identities so tightly, like a security blanket. Any threat to our identity is a threat to us, often triggering a response. We identify ourselves by how we dress—I know I prefer certain brands and styles that make me look and feel a certain way, namely professional, sharp, stylish. Here, that is not an option. Hence my obsession with the white pajamas, which strip away all control over my image.

It's not only our clothes. Out there, we identify ourselves based on our homes and all our stuff inside our four walls. In here, we have a monastic cell, with only a few cherished objects we have brought from home.

We also identify ourselves with what we do. I have for many years. Here, I am consciously not working, so I have temporarily let go of that part of my identity. Others, though, continue to work—sending emails, taking calls, etc. Why? If they can afford to come to a place like this and take two to three weeks away from life, surely they are well established professionally and probably not dependent on their income to survive. But maybe being dependent on work is part of their identity.

Another way we identify ourselves is based on where we are from. It's one of the first questions the doctors ask us—to know the climate we're used to, as well as the culture. "It's complicated" is how I respond when other patients here ask me. "Originally, I'm from Canada. But I have been living in Lisbon, Portugal, for the past few years. Not sure where I'll be spending my time this year, probably some combination of Sydney, where my partner lives, and London. Oh, and my family is originally from Delhi." That last part I add for all the Europeans who see an Indian man in India speaking without an Indian accent.

We identify ourselves through our family and loved ones, too. Some of the older women love to gush about their kids and grandkids, telling me their names, where they live, and their stories. I see so much pride in their faces. But by choosing to be fully offline and turn off my phone for the entire seventeen days, the people, places, and projects I normally rely on for my identity are temporarily out of my conscious mind. In deconstructing these dimensions of identity, I recognize that being here has allowed me to momentarily dissociate with everything, everywhere, and everyone. What's left of me when I remove everything? Who am I without my clothes, my house, my work, my location, and my family? Who is "Kunal"?

Day Eight: Steam Box
Sweating it out

"I like your red sneakers," I say as my opening line while on the walking path this morning. She pauses, looks at me, and returns a smile. "Yes, they are quite bright, aren't they?"

Both dressed in our white pajamas, there is not much else to complement each other on to open a conversation.

"I wore a similar pair like those for five years, every single day. They were a great conversation starter and people always noticed them," I share.

"Yes, there's something unique about bright red shoes. They are a statement, I guess."

As we exchange pleasantries and get to know each other, I learn that Judy is a fellow Canadian, from Vancouver, who arrived the day before. She has two sons, has worked in international development for thirty years, has six horses, runs a business of some sort, and appreciates art very much. She's here for twenty-eight days and seems to having something of a life crisis. I am not sure what's going on; however, I can sense her emotional energy is agitated and low.

We start talking about Kerala, and to distract her, I share more with her about its history, some of which I learned on my first time visiting years back.

Kerala is a state in the southern part of India, known as the "spiritual state." Its lush green landscapes, waterways, and beaches make it a popular domestic and international tourist destination. One of Kerala's distinguishing features is its extensive network of interconnected canals, rivers, lakes, and inlets. These backwaters are home to a variety of flora and fauna, and houseboat tours offer a unique way to experience it, which I did when I visited for the first time.

Kerala boasts the highest literacy rate in all of India, cited as near 100 percent because they prioritize education here. Kerala's economy is supported by a combination of traditional industries like agriculture, fishing, and handicrafts, and modern industries such as tourism, tech, and business process outsourcing.

Certain communities in Kerala follow a matrilineal system, where lineage and inheritance are traced through the female line. Women are central to decision-making in the family, and property passes from mother to daughter. This system stands in contrast to the patriarchal norm prevalent in most other parts of India, and the world.

Historically, in these societies, men were often involved in military campaigns and other travel-related activities, enabling women to take on significant roles in managing properties and family affairs. This system has helped empower women within their communities, ensuring their economic and social security.

Over time, these matrilineal practices have evolved and changed, especially with the influence of modern laws and societal changes. However, the legacy of these practices continues to influence Kerala, making it a distinct and interesting aspect of its cultural heritage.

The predominant language in Kerala is Malayalam, which is quite distinct from Hindi, the language I am fluent in. My efforts to communicate with the staff in any language other than English have not been successful due to the significant differences between Malayalam and Hindi.

I have to pause here in my historical monologue, since Judy has to go to her first ghee treatment. I wish her luck and tell her I look forward to seeing her again soon.

I go on with the usual morning consultation and treatments. First, another four-handed massage. Again, it is intense.

Next is something new: the steam box.

The steam box is a small wooden structure with a small bench inside to sit, and two doors that shut me inside. There is a small, circular cutout at the top for my neck. It looks like I'm sitting in a coffin, or an upright version of one of those boxes magicians use when they saw an assistant in half. It is quite comical to be inside this contraption with only my head popping out.

The steam mechanism is the most interesting part, though. Next to the box is a gas stove, and a good old-fashioned pressure cooker on top with one important modification: a rubber pipe coming out of the cooker lid that feeds the steam box. The stove stays on the entire time, meaning the pressure continues to build in the cooker, sending the steam into the box. And I sit there, like a turkey, steam-cooking inside the box.

The steam is infused with a lemongrass scent that I love. I imagine it isn't an essential oil but actual lemongrass plant inside the pressure cooker. Even the steam has a yellow tint to it, which I can see on my loincloth when I emerge.

Surprisingly, my steam lasts only seven minutes. Compared to hour-long saunas I've taken back home, this is highly effective and efficient. Similar to the advice given after a sauna, I am told to not shower for another two hours, as my body temperature is now quite elevated, and it's best to continue to perspire and release all of the toxins. I feel great the rest of the afternoon and continue to enjoy the lemongrass scent that oozes out of my skin.

Later that evening, after dinner, I run into Judy again on the walking path, still in her white pajamas. This time, she opens up a bit more.

She is sixty-three years old and has had a rough couple of years. A serious accident, divorce, diagnosis of multiple sclerosis, debilitating pain, surgery after surgery, and still, no signs of getting better. In addition to the physical suffering she has endured, I sense the worst of it is emotional. For the first time in her life, she is not a high-functioning person, and that has hit her identity hard. She worries about how her sons will see her and wants to be there for them. She worries about her business. She worries a lot about what she will think of herself if she fails.

As I listen to her story and struggles, I empathize with her for the journey she's going through. I see that sharing all of this, with a stranger, is starting to lift some of the emotional weight, if only for a while. But that is a start.

At one point later in our walk, she says, "I'm tired of trying so hard."

We both let out a big sigh. And then laugh. I share her frustration completely and have at many times felt the same. She asks if I also have been a productivity-junkie, always trying to be useful and contributing to society, my world, or my life.

"Yes. All. The. Time."

That's all I have to offer—not advice but being able to relate.

As we part ways for the evening, my impulse to say something leads to me say, "I hope you figure out how to not try so hard." She smiles. Then I add, "And then you can teach me." She laughs, and we hug each other goodnight.

Day Nine: Purgation
Nothing left to hold

Today is purgation day. Ever since I learned that ghee, massage, and other practices aren't the main event, I have been dreading purgation most of all the panchakarma treatments. My morning meditation has been helpful to calm my nerves and remind me that discomfort is part of the process here. Discomfort is to be expected, not to be feared or avoided.

I have been told that my prescribed purgation is induced diarrhea. Earlier today Patrick told me that he went to the toilet twenty times on purgation day. He seemed quite jolly about that because he had heard of others having to go thirty times. It's all about perspective, I guess.

I had a colonoscopy a few years ago, and the preparation for that treatment felt like a purgation of sorts—my colon was definitely empty by the end. They didn't find anything in the colonoscopy, thankfully; however, I noticed that the preparation actually had a lot of benefit after the fact. That was the last time I had induced diarrhea—and it was mild compared to what was ahead.

Today there are no steamed apples at breakfast and no water in the morning. I go to the treatment building at 8:00 a.m. and see the doctor. He wears a big smile on his face. I don't. He explains that the purpose of purgation isn't to clean the colon, as it had been in my colonoscopy procedure. Rather, the purpose of purgation in the context of panchakarma is to support the digestive tract in releasing all of the excess toxins that it's been collecting as part of the ghee process. The medicine that induces diarrhea is a combination of herbs. I'm amazed by the sophistication of ancient medicine, and how much can be accomplished with herbs. He gives me a glimmer of hope, though. He says some people only have to release once, while others have to release up to thirty times. He asks me to keep count.

I take the medicine, which tastes as awful as I expect, and slowly make my way back to my room. I am told not to leave my room, as once the medicine starts to work, it could happen anytime. It will be involuntary, he explained, and I am not to be more than a few feet away from the bathroom all day. I am to drink a half glass of warm water every thirty minutes to counteract dehydration and keep things moving.

After one hour, the first release happens. I'll save you the description—but know it is intense. Not painful but forceful, if that makes sense. About thirty minutes later, again. After one more hour, the third evacuation and. after twenty more minutes, a fourth.

At midday the doctor checks on me. I feel vulnerable having him in my space, given what is going on. Despite seeing him a few times a day and developing a rapport with him, it is a new level of intimacy having him step into my room, especially while I am feeling this weak.

His visit lasts only a few minutes, and he then sends some rice porridge for me from the kitchen. I take a few spoons of it, and then comes number five. Followed in quick succession by six, seven, and eight, twenty minutes apart. All from a mouthful of rice! I decide I won't bother trying to eat. My gut is clearly telling me not to.

To keep myself occupied and distracted, I begin reading a book, appropriately called Letting Go. Written by a doctor, it's mostly about the impacts of repressed and suppressed emotions on the body and on life. The author shares techniques for releasing stored emotion and goes into detail about levels of consciousness.

It is absolutely the right book for me to read at this point in the panchakarma process. While my body is releasing, I have the urge to journal constantly about different major life events and the emotions they induced that I still carry. I work through them, page by page, which releases many of the negative feelings I hadn't known I was still holding onto. A lot of important moments in my adult life come up and bring me to tears. Family. Relationships. Friendships. Business. Identity. Everything. By the afternoon, I have used all the tissues in my room to wipe some part of me.

Despite the ache in my gut and depletion of my body, my heart feels at peace and mind at ease. At one moment, a smile appears on my face. It is beautiful. I slowly walk over to my bed, sit on a pillow in my white pajamas, and close my eyes to begin meditating. A rush of positive emotions floods my body. Followed by tears of joy and peace. I forget about my physical pain and discomfort, as I feel connected to something beyond this moment.

As an observer watching my life, I feel compassion for Kunal and the journey he's been on, in particular the past few years. I observe him moving through life, visualizing the places, the people, and the projects that have occupied his attention. I see the moments he felt elated and the moments he felt deflated. I can only smile, sending him love as I connect to his innocence.

After the meditation, I open my journal and begin to write again. This time, a poem flows out. It is in a different tone and structure than most of my writing. It is as if I am being spoken to. Instead of writing as "I," I show up in the poem as "you." The poem is an instruction manual for how to live. How to live in this new state, of having released repressed and stored emotions. How to live with my heart. To me, it is beautiful and inspirational.

I cry again and again and again. Something profound has shifted inside me this afternoon—I can feel it.

The last time I felt this type of shift was ten years ago. I had come to a moment in life where I had everything I wanted professionally and personally, yet felt no joy about that accomplishment. It was the moment when I first turned inward and began to question how to live. It was the moment I began to open up to my own spirituality and, soon after, discovered tools like meditation and yoga, to support my process of discovering how I wanted to live.

It is no surprise, then, that I called my first book How to Live, which was released a few months before this trip to India. In it, I cover the past ten years of my life, from that moment until now. It is full of stories of how I experimented with life, trying to unlearn everything I knew and rediscover myself.

It is only fitting that the release of that book coincides with the release of some long-repressed emotions and toxins that have been hanging around in my gut. Now I have so much more space for a new beginning. It's too early to know what's starting; however, at a deeper level, I do know that my life is about to go through another set of changes, as I relearn how I want to live again. Maybe I will have to revise and reissue How to Live.

The doorbell rings, which brings me back into my physical reality. I answer it to find someone has brought me a glass of coconut water. A broad smile comes onto my face once again. I receive it with a heart full of gratitude and warmth.

The coconut water, like everything else, has a purpose: to replenish the fluids and electrolytes I have been losing all day. It is also the only cool drink I have had since arriving here. I savor each drop, even though shortly after I have movements nine and ten.

Later that evening, dinner is sent to my room. I have no appetite but force myself to eat at least a little, feeling physically weak though spiritually energized and very much alive. Number eleven.

I lie down to sleep around 9:00 p.m., sensing that my life has forever changed. It is a good purgation day.

Day Ten: New Treatments
Pain held gently

I am woken at 04:30 a.m. by the sound of loud chanting from a speaker system. It's coming from outside the hospital grounds.

Kerala is known for its religious diversity, something I witnessed firsthand when I visited last time. The major religions practiced in Kerala are Hinduism, Islam, and Christianity; I remember visiting a building with my father with three floors. The ground floor was a Christian church, the middle floor a Hindu temple, the top floor a mosque. It was inspiring to see the acceptance and integration of different religions in one physical place. That building is an inspiration for how the world could live in greater harmony.

Kerala is home to some of the oldest and most famous Hindu temples in India. Islam in Kerala also has a long history, dating back to the time of the Prophet Muhammad. The state has a significant Muslim population, and they celebrate festivals like Eid.

Kerala's coastal cities have historical significance in the spread of Islam in the region.

Christianity in Kerala is believed to have been introduced in the first century AD. Kerala has a significant Christian population, and the state is known for its ancient churches, Syrian Christian community, and distinctive Christian traditions.

Having now remembered that I'm in a place that celebrates, very loudly, all its religions, I crawl out of bed to begin my morning routine of meditation, journaling, walking, yoga, and breakfast. My own religion.

I receive a plate full of fresh papaya at breakfast today. The bright orange fruit is juicy and replenishing. I normally don't eat too much fruit, as I notice it leads to blood sugar spikes . . . and then crashes. When I told the doctor this in our first meeting, he said, "Let's see what happens." After eating a plate full of fruit, I go for a gentle walk, and back in my room by 07:30 a.m., I fall back asleep.

I wake up in a blissful haze, rested and peaceful, with my mind calm but my body weak, (no surprise, given how little I have eaten and how much water I lost in the past twenty-four hours). Slowly, I make my way slowly to the treatment building for the morning consultation.

Remembering the day I had yesterday—in particular the emotional release, spiritual inspiration, and mental clarity—I notice a lightness and ease in my step. As I pass by other patients, dressed in their white pajamas, I smile more. While waiting for the doctor, one of the other patients even remarks, "You look happy!" I am in a new state of heightened consciousness—aware of so much more outside and inside of me. And receiving all of it with a smile from my heart.

After the usual routine of questions and answers, the doctor takes a little longer listening to my pulse on my right wrist. I asked him what changed. I had been asking him about my pulse each morning, to which he would laugh and say, "I'll tell you after purgation." Well, it is after purgation now, so I am eager to find out.

"It's much different today," he remarks, finally giving me an answer, still not clear about how it's different, though.

"What changed?" I ask more pointedly. He shares that my pulse has become more rhythmic. During the ghee therapy, he says, my pulse reacted in all sorts of different ways and was highly inconsistent. I don't get much more from him; however, he seems pleased with the progress of my pulse. Good enough for me.

Today is a turning point in the quantity of treatments I receive.

First treatment of the day: drinking a liquid that is meant to increase my immunity. As they bring the tray close to me, I see the chaser of warm water and a napkin—a signal that this isn't going to taste good. I'm right.

Second treatment: two short, scrawny men oil my naked body from head to toe. Not a square inch of my body is left unoiled. Then, armed with pouches full of leaves that have been soaked in boiling water, they pat me firmly and rhythmically all over for one hour. Every ten minutes, I am told to change position, be it on my front, back, or side (my favorite), or sitting up. Since there are two of them, it's more like a two-hour-long beating. I hope this is the closest I'll ever be to being actually beaten up. It is a vulnerable and humbling position to be in. The massage is not focused on the muscles but on releasing the toxins in the uppermost layers of skin. The oil binds to the toxins that are being beaten out of me. By the end, I'm surprised by how relaxed I feel.

Third treatment: the application of oil to clear my sinuses and facial skin, and support brain health. The doctor comes back into the room for this one, a sign it is more serious. I'm lying on my back and still oily after the beating treatment, now wearing a loin cloth. The doctor has a small dropper bottle in his hand. He squirts about ten drops of the oil in my right nostril, asks me to inhale deeply through that same nostril, sending the oil deeper into my sinus cavity, and then exhale through my mouth. Same thing on the other side.

And then the gross part. I sit up and cough up the mucus or any remaining oil. This is followed by a warm water gargle. Then I am told to lie back down, at which time the therapist waves a boiling-hot cloth in front of my face as a steamer, to make sure the oil doesn't solidify. Then I sit back up, repeat the spitting and gargling routine, lie back down, and do it all again. After four times, I'm done.

As I walk out of the treatment room, the doctor sees me off and reminds me not to blow my nose for at least one hour. I innocently ask him how many times I'd be doing that treatment. He says, "At least three times, and then after that we'll see."
My face drops.

I am bored today, for the first time here.
This is the longest stretch of time in my adult life I've been disconnected from my professional world, including my devices, my inbox, my text messages, my stock portfolio. But it's also the longest stretch without communicating with my parents, my sister, my friends. It is the longest I've gone without video calls with my three-year-old nephew since he was born.
I feel fortunate to be able to disconnect during this experiment—it has helped me with all aspects of the detox. I'm the only patient here who is fully disconnected. Though I can't know what the others are experiencing, I sense that without the distractions of work and home the detox for me is much more intense.

The disconnection is worth it because it's working. I am pleasantly surprised how the quality of my passive thoughts has changed since I arrived. Without the stimulus and influx of information that I constantly triage into meaningful and meaningless categories, I notice that I'm engaging in more calm, quiet, and peaceful introspection.

I am living outside time. Wearing the same white pajamas each day, passing by the same fellow patients along the walking paths, seeing the same therapist twice a day, the same staff members around the grounds, there is a regularity to it all that makes me feel the world has come to a standstill. There are no visible indicators that time has progressed. I forget what day of the week it is, or day of the month. I have to think hard to work out what month and year it is. None of that matters in the present moment.

Day Eleven: Beyond Thought
The space between

A new day, another new treatment. Today is the "forehead oil drip" treatment—a unique and unexpected experience.

The treatment starts as most do: stripping down, putting on a loin cloth, and getting oiled up from head to toe by two short Indian men. Then, once I am on my back, the therapists guide my head into a precise position under a metal bowl hanging from a delicate stand. It takes a solid few minutes of tiny adjustments to make sure my head is exactly where it needs to be.

Once again, the doctor comes back into the room . . . so, this is serious. He explains to me what is going to happen in very few words, raising more questions than answers in my mind. Today, I don't prod for more explanation; I just close my eyes and trust the process. The doctor leaves, which is a relief, and the therapists place cotton balls on my eyes and a thin cloth headband above my eyebrows. The anticipation grows as I wait to feel something.

At first, it feels like a paintbrush saturated with hot oil is gliding back and forth across my forehead. Then I feel the oil start to stream back over my forehead into my hair. Then the oil steadily drips onto my forehead, and it glides to cover my entire forehead and slides into my hair. It's like nothing else I've felt before.

I focus on my breath and relax into the treatment. I wonder how long I'll be here. At first, the sensation all over my forehead makes it hard to think about anything else. I had prepared myself to fall into a meditative state; however, the newness of the experience prevents me from going there right away. Over time, my mind settles and the tranquil experience I expected arrives.

My thoughts wander to the destinations I'm used to visiting in meditation. And then I fall asleep, dreaming about missing planes and running through airports. After waking from my nap, I realize where I am, and that the hot oil is still painting my forehead. Surprisingly, there is no oil in my eyes or ears; all the fussing over my head's position at the start was worth it. I notice that, at times, the oil feels cool; at times, warm. I doubt the temperature of the oil is actually changing; it's my experience that's changing. The treatment goes on for one hour.

Afterwards, I am relaxed and calm, like I have stepped into a different dimension of myself. There are no strong thoughts filling my mind.

I am not to wash my hair for at least three hours and must not to use any shampoo when I do. They tie a cloth around my head, and as I walk the grounds, I see everyone wearing a cloth covering their hair. We all had the treatment today.

It's the first time I am able to attend the daily yoga nidra class. My first time doing yoga nidra was in Bali five years ago, and, despite having done thousands of yoga and meditation classes in my lifetime so far, I still remember this specific class. The experience was powerful.

Yoga nidra, often referred to as "yogic sleep," is a practice that brings the practitioner to the threshold of waking and sleeping consciousness. It is more like meditation than the physical movement practice that most people think of as yoga in the West. Through guided instructions, the practitioner moves through stages of relaxation with full, conscious awareness for systematic relaxation of the body, breath awareness, and the exploration of sensory and emotional thought patterns. The destination is a profound state of relaxation and inner stillness, while maintaining a trace of awareness.

Unlike regular sleep, where we lose consciousness, yoga nidra allows one to stay in a state of semi-awareness. This state is beneficial for reducing stress and anxiety, enhancing creativity, improving sleep quality, and overall wellbeing. It's a gentle yet powerful practice that can help balance the nervous system and release deeply held tensions in the mind and body.

After my yogic sleep, I feel an even deeper shift in my awareness. It's getting closer to night, but I feel lighter and more awake. Each practice today has supported this progression.

As I leave the yoga hall in my white pajamas and walk back to my room, I notice for the first time the flowers blooming all around me. The red, orange, green, and yellow petals shine brightly in the moonlight. I hear the birds and admire their colorful feathers. I lock eyes with one long enough to take in its blue feathers, yellow beak, tiny feet, and round black eyes—as if I am taking a photo in my mind. The birds here are calm, I notice, unlike the frenetic city bids I'm used to avoiding.

Another smile spreads across my face. There are no other thoughts in my mind.

Day Twelve: Namaste
To see and be seen

While waiting for my consultation today, a middle-aged Austrian woman in her white pajamas next to me strikes up a conversation. We debrief about our day, and I learn about a water treatment she had for inflammation management and alleviating stiffness in the joints. It sounds intense.

It consisted of her lying on her back, on the wooden massage table, while two therapists dripped medicated water over her body from brass bottles continuously—for nearly an hour. Her mind went all over the place during that hour. At times, it felt like she was swimming in the ocean. At other times, like she was in a womb.

She told me she experiences quite a bit of physical pain in her shoulders, lower back, and knees. When her sciatic nerve is aggravated, it sends pain through her lower back and down her leg; when it happens, she can't lie still for more than an hour without needing to move. So, when she's asleep at night, her body moves, although it's subtle enough that it usually doesn't wake her. At least, not to the point of consciousness.

Hearing her experience, my heart swells with empathy and compassion for those who are living with chronic pain and discomfort. I admire her grace and calm despite her situation, as well as her courage to come to such a hospital to try and alleviate it.

Later in the day, I catch up with a new friend walking along the path in his white pajamas. He is an Indian man who has been living in London the past twenty years. He is a jolly fellow, striking up conversation with everyone throughout the stay, always smiling and laughing. When I ask him if he'll be returning to the hospital some time, he responds, "I hope I don't have to."

It transpires that the past year has been quite stressful for him. As a result, he's gained over twenty pounds—a lot of weight to put on in one year. His blood pressure has also been rising. He felt he needed a jolt, something intense, to help him get back onto a healthy living track. His goal was to lose around fifteen pounds during his twenty-one-day stay.

"How's it going so far?" I inquire.

"I lost 11 pounds in the first week. And I'm getting closer to my goal. It feels great."

He glows with pride and health. The initial few pounds were from water retention and relatively easy to lose, he explains; however, the diet, the treatments, and the walking (especially the walking) have helped him reverse his weight-gain trend. I admire his strength and determination.

His friend, who had encouraged him to come, had lost 26 pounds in his first visit, and another 15 in his second visit, one year later.

I think back to the caution I was given about sharing our treatments and protocols with other patients. I've been eating a ton—and maybe gained a few needed pounds—yet the same Ayurveda is being used for the complete opposite with other patients here. Amazing how the basic principles of movement, rest, and healthy eating can help a body find its own state of health and homeostasis.

Next is the yoga session: pranayama. After the exercises, I sit in meditation for a bit longer, hoping to build on the heightened sense of inner awareness I have been feeling the past few days. I start to recap the many conversations I had in the day with other patients and again feel empathy and compassion for how each of us are following our own health journeys with integrity here.

I also realize that this place feeds my introverted side. From the eating in silence, to the silent yoga practice a few different times per day, and the silent massages. They encourage us, despite our best efforts, to minimize conversations with one another. Even though at times it feels isolating, I'm enjoying the space to be silent.

When I see the doctor next, I share that I have noticed for years that my stomach seems to have a mild sensitivity to . . . everything. The first few bites of most meals trigger some digestive discomfort.

"Chew your food twenty to thirty times before swallowing—every single bite. I know it's hard, but you will see, it will make a difference," he says.

At lunch, I try just that. And my stomach doesn't say anything. At dinner, I have two servings, which take me forty-five minutes to eat with this excessive chewing strategy, when normally I'd finish the meal in ten to fifteen minutes. I am the last one left in the dining hall. And again, similar to lunch, no reaction from my stomach.

I'm feeling encouraged—and inspired.

One surprisingly sweet ritual here is that everyone greets each other by pressing their hands in a prayer position, the gesture of greeting known as namaste (the gesture often accompanied by saying the word "namaste") every time there is an interaction, no matter how small or large.

When I walk into the treatment hall, the doctor welcomes me with namaste, I do the same. The other doctors who are waiting for their patients that make eye contact with me also greet me with namaste. I do the same. The therapist greets me with namaste at the start and end of the treatment. I do the same. While walking to the therapy room, I pass half a dozen therapists waiting for their patients, and each greets me with namaste. I do the same.

After the daily treatment, I walk a few circuits of the path. The garden women cleaning the leaves that had fallen the previous day greet me with namaste. I do the same. The garden men watering the endless variety of trees greet me with namaste. I do the same.

After my walk, I go to the dining hall for lunch. The staff greets me with namaste, when I arrive and when I leave. I do the same. After lunch on my way back to my room, I pass another patient in her white pajamas. We each greet one another with namaste.

Like this, it continues. I easily namaste at least one hundred times a day here. It's special and quite something to see how the energy of a place shifts when everyone makes eye contact, smiles, and adds a physical gesture to say, "I see you"—the essence of the meaning of this gesture. And to see it reciprocated is to feel seen. And to feel seen is really what we all are looking for in life, isn't it?

Day Thirteen: The Mosquito
Surrendering control

After dinner last night, I felt inspired to re-read one of my favorite books of all time: Siddhartha, by Herman Hesse.

I first read Siddhartha ten years ago, as I was beginning to develop my meditation practice and open up to my own spirituality. I had already read a few books about Buddhism and the story of the Buddha, however Siddhartha is an alternative perspective with the same underlying message. Written more than a hundred years ago, originally in German, it is a well-known classic amongst spiritual seekers.

It's a short read, so I whipped through half of it between dinner and bedtime. The writing is so descriptive that my dreams involved the characters. I felt I was there, two thousand years ago, observing the story and imagining the scenes. Although it's been at least five years since I last re-read Siddhartha, my subconscious dreaming mind remembered the story and sequence of scenes in the whole book. It's fascinating what the subconscious stores.

This morning in meditation, sitting quietly and peacefully cross-legged on my bed in my white pajamas, I hear a buzzing sound. A mosquito has joined me for meditation. My instinct is to swat it away or squash it. I've killed a dozen, maybe two dozen, mosquitos since arriving, and yet have as many bites on my limbs and neck.

This morning, though, my instinct feels different. Instead of wanting to swat it away or kill it, I begin to connect with the mosquito and try to communicate with it in my mind. Instead of leading with fearful thoughts like "please don't bite me" or "leave me alone," or angry thoughts like "you'd better not bite me," I try encouragement: "There's something more interesting for you over there than over here." Offering a carrot, instead of a stick.

I then have the spontaneous urge to name the mosquito. I call it Frank. The moment it has an identity, I have an uneasy sensation in my stomach at the thought of killing Frank. By personifying the mosquito, I can relate to it and want to show it kindness, not violence.

Then my mind goes to a place of acceptance. If Frank bites me, that's okay. I can handle it; he's just responding to its biological response to obtain nutrients, not trying to harm me. Frank's brothers and sisters have already bitten me anyway. It was a reminder that my body can tolerate uncomfortable and irritating sensations. And if my body can, so can my mind.

The next thing I hear is my meditation timer ring. My thirty-five-minute morning meditation ritual is complete, and Frank has not bitten me. At least not yet. I feel like there's been a software upgrade in my mind. One that leads with positive thinking and manifestation. Inspired by my reading and reflecting, I have a new impulse to lead with what I desire, versus what I fear. It sends the desired vibration into the universe. It also helps me feel more at ease.

At yoga this morning, I newly appreciate how simple and gentle the poses are. Designed to bolster the Ayurvedic treatments, they are the supporting actors, not the stars. Despite this, their effect is powerful. The before-and-after effect I feel from simple guided exercises is dramatic. A reminder of the power of subtle changes.

In Western culture, we mostly encourage force, power, and strength. I've been steeped in Western yoga culture for ten years and have done nearly one thousand classes in at least a dozen countries. The "no pain, no gain" mantra has dominated my experience of yoga, with the emphasis often on pushing ourselves to reach new heights. My conditioning has taught me to think, If it doesn't feel challenging, then there must not be any benefit.

Learning to practice yoga here is different. Although it is practiced in such a peaceful, gentle, restorative, and calm manner, I still feel strong, powerful, flexible, and able in my body. This has opened my eyes, and I now understand why the practices have stood the test of time over thousands of years.

I now understand why they say yoga is accessible to everyone. It is not about being flexible in the body but about being flexible in the mind. It is not a performative, competitive sport, like it may seem if one looks at social media or attends yoga studios in New York or Los Angeles. But yoga should be a personalized practice, meant to serve your own body. I used to try to get my body to do whatever the instructor asked us to do, or, more honestly, what the person on the mat next to mine was able to do. That was all about my ego. Being able to do complex, and sometimes dangerous, Instagram-worthy yoga poses and compete with the other students in class never makes my body feel good, even though it may make my mind feel good.

Over the years, and especially here at the hospital, as I have felt more connected to my body and developed the skills to listen to it rather than directing and controlling it, my practice has evolved to incorporate the poses my body needs. If my shoulders are tight, I'll do shoulder stretches. If my neck is sore on one side, I'll hold a pose for an extended amount of time on that side. If my legs are stiff, I'll do some lunges. If my lower back is sensitive, I'll do abdominal exercises. Minimal effort, maximum results.

The word yoga translates to "union." And my experience of yoga is that it can be used to help connect me with my own body and its needs.

Today I receive another one of the five panchakarma treatments: enema. It all happens very quickly. After another forehead oil treatment, the doctor walks into the room. He asks me to lie on my side, bend one leg and breathe through my mouth. Then, within about seven seconds, the treatment is done. He injects 100 mL of oil, medicated with herbs, into my rectum. "Finished," the doctor announces before swiftly leaving the room.

As the therapist sits me up, to get me ready for my post-treatment shower, I feel a new level of vulnerability as I realize that he has now seen more parts of my body than I ever will.

Walking through the gardens back to my room, I try to sense any response to the enema treatment, but I feel nothing. This suggests to me that so much of our experience is in the mind and that my body can handle much more than I give it credit for. My mind is the fearful one, often getting in the body's way of health and healing.

Day Fourteen: Passion
Play without pressure

Today during the morning consultation, the doctor checks my weight. I have lost 6 pounds since arriving, an effect of these detox treatments. That is unexpected. I don't need to lose weight, if anything I could use a few extra pounds.

Most people have had their weight checked in the past day or two, and everyone is enthusiastic about their weight loss. My German friend, Patrick, who has taken a liking to me, shares that he lost 17 pounds the last time he was here and is on track for something similar. Another patient is delighted she has lost 11 pounds already.

I believe some of the initial weight loss is due to the massages. They are stimulating and thorough, and after each one, I find that I urinate quite a bit, despite not having had much water beforehand. I also believe some of it is the food. The ingredients are fresh, everything is cooked within one hour of serving, and the quantity of food is strictly managed, preventing overeating and cravings.

I also believe the walking is key. With few other activities to occupy our time, people are easily covering five or six miles a day. I have not been as active walking here, as I'm not trying to lose weight; however, for those who are, it is clearly working.

Perhaps, also, some of the weight-loss success is aided by the loosely fitted white pajamas. With fewer inhibitions, we can all relax a bit, which is allowing our bodies to let go of even more.

Today I realized that this whole experience is particularly meaningful for me, as I identify as Indian. Most of the others are European, who see being in India as a novelty. For me, it's a way to connect with my own culture. I recognize the subtleties that non-Indians may not pick up on so easily, be it the namaste greetings, or the reason we wear slippers not "outside shoes," or why the priest chants prayers and sounds the bell at specific times of the day. I better understand the religious symbols carved into the columns of some of the buildings and the interactions with the doctor and therapists, beyond the head nodding, and the chants at the start and end of each yoga and pranayama class, and the hand-washing ritual at the start and end of each meal. I can empathize with the staff members, able to determine with just one look what their class status is and if they are educated. I can see the hidden hierarchy.

After breakfast today I meet Olena from Ukraine, walking along the path. She's forty-two, and it's her third visit to the hospital in three years. I initiate conversation with her, and we quickly dig into philosophizing, skipping the pleasantries and usual ice-breaker topics when meeting someone new. Enlightenment. Soul. Purpose. Meditation. Reincarnation. We really get into it. As the topics continue to unravel, our walking speed seems to accelerate as we make round after round on the path and in our conversation.

I learn that, four years ago, she left her family business after ten years of working there, as she realized it was not meaningful for her. She left without knowing what was next. I admire her courage and can relate. In the few months of "nothingness," as she described it, one day she decided to become a pianist.

"Hold on, back up here. Tell me, where did this inspiration come from? Did you play as a child?"

"Nope, I had never once played the piano. I didn't know a single person who played or even owned a piano. I was listening to someone playing on the radio one day and just felt a spark. I thought that I'd like to be able to play like that."

She has spent the past four years learning to become a pianist and was recently named the number-one pianist internationally in her category. She practices full-time, six to eight hours a day, and will often play for four hours continuously, without pause. She became a pianist. Seemingly, out of nowhere.

However, yesterday, here at the hospital, likely as a result of the environment and the treatments, she realized that in trying to become an exceptional pianist, she'd lost contact with what she loved so much about playing music: the feel of the keys, the sound of the mistaken and out-of-place notes, the surprise of not knowing what a new song sheet might sound like. In her ambition to succeed at being a pianist, she forgot why she chose to get started in the first place.

It is an important reminder: do not let a passion become a profession. As a businessman, I've long believed that there is a fine line between passion and profession, and once a passion becomes a profession, then we can easily lose the passion. Olena's story is an example of this.

Writing is my passion—I really do love it. I started journaling ten years ago and write privately almost daily. I also have been writing publicly on a blog for about ten years and, in the past four years, have published every Sunday without fail. Last year, I drafted three books, published one of them, and the other two are about to be released. What you're reading will be my fourth.

However, after the launch of my first book a few months ago, I started to pay more attention to the promotion and distribution of my books, including talking with others who self-publish about what they learned, doing online research, listening to podcasts, and more. I stopped writing and got caught up in the business of publishing.

Here at the hospital, I've been writing a lot in my private journal, and I'm sure this has helped me release emotion, which has had a positive impact on my physical wellbeing. It has been the perfect environment for me to dive deep into my passion for writing and use it as a form of expression, using writing as a vehicle for sharing more of myself, especially with those close to me.

Olena's love for piano, my love for writing: I believe it's healthy to have a passion that allows us to express ourselves—and to keep it a passion to avoid making it a profession.

Day Fifteen: The Food
Tasting simplicity

By now, you may have noticed I've hardly mentioned details about the food at the hospital. This is intentional—mostly to tease my parents, as I know the first question they'll ask me when I come home is about the food. My response will be, "You don't go to a hospital like this for the food!" However, in this hospital, of course, food is part of the medicine.

Fifteen days in, I can now confirm that the hospital really does treat food as medicine—because it's delicious. I understand how food is a core part of the healing process. The food is all cooked, nothing is raw, except the occasional fruit sampling. Everything is easy to digest, as the food is prepared to support the treatments. And we're all feeling better after eating it.

Today I get chatty with one of the dining hall staff about Ayurvedic food. I ask him how old he is, guessing mid-twenties.

"Thirty-six years old, sir," he replies with a downward glance.

"What? No way!" I remark, genuinely shocked.

He has been working with this Ayurvedic hospital for sixteen years. Which means he has been eating this food, cooked in this way, for all that time—as the staff eat the same food as the guests. That must be the secret to his youthfulness.

He shares with me part of the Kerala approach to food is to have big lunches and light dinners. Everything is about digestion in Ayurveda, and you'll see that the locals eat very small dinners, always with only cooked food. That often means salads in the evening. This approach is also found throughout the culture. For example, weddings happen during the daytime, with lunch being the main meal. The dishes at the hospital are inspired by the local cuisine. Kerala has a distinctive cuisine that mirrors its multicultural history, abundant natural resources, and the tropical climate—it's completely different from the rich, heavy North Indian cuisine I grew up with.

One of the hallmark ingredients in Kerala cuisine is coconut. Given the abundance of coconut trees in the region, grated coconut and its milk are widely used in various dishes, leaving a unique flavor and texture. Here, coconut oil is also the primary cooking oil, unlike North Indian cuisine, where ghee or vegetable oils are more commonly used.

For example, yesterday I tried confirming with the doctor that the chutney wasn't made with yogurt, as I have a lactose sensitivity. He was confused by my question, and kept responding, "It's chutney." After the back-and-forth, he finally got why I was asking. "You won't find any yogurt used in any Kerala chutneys, anywhere here in the South," he said. Apparently, that's only done in the North.

Kerala's trade history means that spices like black pepper, cardamom, cloves, ginger, and cinnamon are used generously, often freshly ground. The flavors tend to be more subtle yet rich, compared to the often bold and hearty flavors in North Indian dishes created by using turmeric, asafetida, cumin, and powdered mango. The spice and salt levels are extremely low at the hospital— surprisingly, I've gotten used to it.

Kerala cuisine features a variety of fermented foods as well, such as appam (a type of pancake made with fermented rice batter and coconut milk) and tapioca.

Ayurveda emphasizes the use of fresh, seasonal ingredients and balancing the six tastes (sweet, sour, salty, pungent/spicy, bitter, and astringent) in every meal. This approach to nutrition is more pronounced in Kerala cuisine than in North Indian cuisine, where the meals are not necessarily created for health as much as flavor.

While North Indian cuisine has a rich array of both vegetarian and non-vegetarian dishes, Kerala cuisine offers an extensive variety of vegetarian options due to its large Hindu population. Meals may be served on a banana leaf during festivals and special occasions. However, Christian and Muslim influences have also made meat and fish popular in parts of the region, and Kerala's long coastline means that seafood is a staple part of the diet in coastal communities. Fish, shrimp, and other seafood are prepared in various ways. There's no seafood here at the hospital, though.

Rice is the staple grain, much more predominant than in North India, where wheat-based breads like naan and roti are more common.

Desserts in Kerala are often rice or coconut-based, like payasam (a sweet dish made of rice, coconut milk, sugar, and spices). North Indian sweets, on the other hand, are typically milk-based, like rasgulla or gulab jamun. Not surprisingly, there are no desserts offered at the hospital.

Despite my family culture, I have come to prefer South Indian cuisine, I think because of the mindful preparation and combination of ingredients. I rarely feel stuffed or bloated after a South Indian meal, the way I often feel after a North Indian meal. I've felt inspired to incorporate more Ayurvedic food principles in my daily life, especially eating cooked foods and using spices.

My relationship with food and physical health has evolved during my stay here. If I'm honest with myself, my motivation to invest in my health over the past few years has been from a place of guilt. This came to me in a journaling session today.

For my entire adult life, I have deprioritized and ignored my physical health, and my body, choosing to be driven by my mind and ego. This involved eating poorly, flying often, no regular exercise, treating sleep as optional, and not listening to my body. Over the years, I started noticing an increase in respiratory illness, and sensing my immune system was struggling I started to change. However, the main motivation for the occasional health drive was guilt—I felt I had to "make up" for not giving my body the attention it needed.

This isn't a healthy way to approach health. Through guilt, I have sometimes made myself feel more unhealthy in the pursuit of health, including intense yoga and creating my pharmacy full of supplements. Furthermore, I've placed expectations on my body of how it needs to perform and function as a result of my investment of time and money into it.

It's like having an old car that is aging and falling apart. One day, you wake up and feel guilty for not taking better care of the car, so you over-invest in repairing all the broken parts at once. Given how much effort I'm putting into repairing this old car, my expectations are now that it will run perfectly—forever. This is the transactional way I've related to my living, breathing, feeling body. A "give and get" mindset.

In the past few weeks, having the space to be with my body and witness its struggle at times with various treatments, I no longer have expectations of it to perform for me. I accept my body as it is. I know it will continue to change. I know it will at times feel weak. At times it will feel strong. And that's okay. I am learning to love my body unconditionally.

The timeless teaching from the Bhagavad Gita, a text at the heart of yoga philosophy written thousands of years ago, is that while everyone has the duty to put in effort, no one has the right to the fruits of their efforts. This is a fitting reminder for me as I make an effort to love, accept, and care for my body without expectation of any specific outcome, and continue to do so after I leave the comfort of the hospital.

Day Sixteen: Childlike
A hand to hold

As my time here is coming to an end, I am starting to feel both sorrow and joy. Sorry to leave this space of healing, but joy to re-enter my world. What I appreciate most about this experience is being taken care of. When I journal about it this morning, it brings me to tears, yet again.

Although I'm a grown adult, I feel more like a child today. Someone else chooses what I wear each day: white pajamas. Someone else chooses what I eat for each meal, and a team of people cook, serve, and clean up after every meal. Someone else chooses which yoga postures and pranayama exercises I will do for the day. Someone else decides what medicine I will have. Someone else oils and massages my body. Someone else cleans my room.

I appreciate not having to make any decisions for myself. It's one thing to take a break from making decisions for my businesses by simply taking a vacation by disconnecting from devices. But even on a regular vacation, I have to choose where to go, what activities to plan, which restaurants to eat at. Not here. It's completely different to have such a limited number of decisions to make daily for my own existence. The last time I was so lacking in responsibility was when I was a child.

Similar to my parents, the people taking care of me here have a lot of love, compassion, empathy, and care. No question I ask the doctor about my body, or about Ayurveda, is too dumb or silly. Any request I have for the therapist, like today's "let's not oil my face," is received generously. This is a hospital that also provides hospitality.

The physical environment here at the hospital makes me feel like a child in a playground. I have not shared too much about it until now, as it was never my focus and should not be a reason why anyone chooses panchakarma at this specific hospital. However, the grounds are inspiring.

As I shared previously, the building itself was built in the fifteenth century. The palace grounds were relandscaped between 2000 and 2003 by the hospital owners to support the Ayurvedic principles of healing. There are hundreds of trees, each with a placard that explains the medicinal healing properties of that tree, alongside its name and origin. The walking path is designed to take the patient on a tour through the many plants that are being used in the medicated oils, ghees, and treatments. Although I won't remember many of their names, I find myself reading the signs by the trees, like walking through an art gallery. This is nature's gallery. It is also a fitting reminder that nature has all the ingredients we need to heal.

I've been exploring deeper layers of consciousness and expanding my awareness over the past week here, with the support of philosophy, meditation, reflection, and yoga. The fact that the environment takes care of all the basic needs, and then some, has been a big contributing factor to my own development and growth. I feel humble and grateful to so many, for so much.

The immersive retreat experience here has also inspired me to do another vipassana meditation retreat. Vipassana is a ten-day silent meditation program that is offered around the world. I have done it a few times now, the last time in 2016. Although I've thought about doing it again since then, more than a few times, I've told friends who would bring it up from time to time, "I'm not feeling it." In truth, I was intimidated.

Despite having done it successfully, and benefited from it greatly, a few times, it was by far the most challenging thing I'd ever done. It takes a lot of strength and courage to sit with your own thoughts, for ten hours a day, for ten days straight, without any distractions or escape outlets. Something like that builds a lot of strength and courage. My time here at the hospital has given me the strength and courage to do another vipassana course, hopefully later this year. I've confronted my mind from a new route, via the body, and have experienced moments of spaciousness and gratitude after releasing so much through my tissues, my sweat, and other places.

The entire panchakarma experience has given me a lot of strength that I can feel at a physical, mental, emotional, and spiritual level. The strength to face parts of myself, and my identity, that I have shied away from. The strength to surrender to the doctor, therapists, and chef, following their instructions without objection. The strength to question and challenge my own beliefs and motivations, in health and in li

I'm curious to see how this enhanced feeling of strength manifests in my life in the coming days, weeks, months, and years. Though I'm not attached to the outcome, I have a strong sense it will be noticeable.

Day Seventeen: Total Transformation

Letting go

This morning as I put on my white pajamas for the last time, a smile spontaneously appears on my face. I did it.

My business brain takes an inventory of my first panchakarma:

108 walking rounds on the hospital campus

85 pages of writing in my journal

34 yoga and pranayama classes

32 Kerala lunches and dinners

29 degrees Celsius, average temperature

23 oil massages

21 fellow patients

17 doctor consultations

11 immune decoctions

6 new friends with whom I hope to stay in touch

6 books read

6 pounds of weight lost

5 ghee drinking treatments

5 nasal drip treatments with medicated oil

5 oil forehead dripping treatments

4 enemas

2 steam box experiences

2 pairs of bamboo slippers worn out

1 panchakarma cleanse and detox completed

Oh, and 17 days of wearing nothing but white pajamas

My white pajamas have evolved to become much more than a uniform. Putting on white pajamas and taking off my normal clothes was symbolic of putting aside my identity, even if temporarily. It is me giving myself permission to be whomever and however I need to be at this moment.

Putting on white pajamas represents commitment to taking someone else's lead—to let someone else make decisions for me and take care of me. It has been a total surrender, a slow letting go of control and any desire to shape my experience.

Putting on white pajamas means I am the same as everyone else here—no better, no worse. I belong here, as does everyone else. There is no space for comparison, we are all unique, even though we dress the same.

Putting on white pajamas was an invitation to become curious, to learn more about Ayurveda, panchakarma,

Kerala, and the south of India. I was shown aspects of my own culture that I had never known before.

Putting on white pajamas was a constant reminder that the purpose of my visit is to heal—body, mind, and spirit. It is not the purpose to be productive in any other dimension of life. It was not to make friends. There is a clear purpose, and I achieved it. I decide to not take home a pair of the hospital's white pajamas in the end, but I feel like I'll be wearing them for the rest of my life.

The benefits of panchakarma and the Ayurvedic retreat environment are already visible to me. Physically, I have lost a few pounds. My stomach is flatter. My body is more flexible. My hair is darker, shinier, and wavier. My eyes are glossy. My skin is smooth, moist, thick, and beautiful, all over. My breathing is deeper. My digestion feels invincible. My sleep has been sound. And I could go on. My body feels better than it did seventeen years ago, let alone seventeen days.

Mentally and emotionally, I also feel lighter. I have let go of deep-seated feelings that I had repressed. I have let go of parts of my identity that are no longer relevant. I have let go of fears, doubts, and insecurities about health, wealth, and relationships. I am determined to adopt more mindfulness into my daily lifestyle. I have been inspired by Ayurvedic food, cooking, and eating principles.

Spiritually and energetically, I feel connected to something bigger than myself. I have learned to place my trust and faith in something greater than me and my actions. To understand that my thoughts manifest my reality—and to choose kind, loving, and positive thoughts over ones filled with fear and insecurity. I feel there is a clear purpose in my life again.

These are some of the benefits I feel today, on day seventeen. However, in speaking with my fellow patients who have returned multiple times, including a Brazilian woman who's here on her twelfth annual visit and looks amazing, the real benefits don't appear until a few weeks and months afterwards.

It is inspiring to remember in modern society that instant gratification isn't nature's way. The benefits I will experience won't end once I leave now that I have put myself on a path of healing. In compiling these reflections of my experience, I found a constructive outlet to direct some of my energy that wasn't consumed by the panchakarma treatments.

Writing has helped me be an observer of my experience, able to appreciate, integrate, share, and derive meaning from it. This is what makes life beautiful: learning to appreciate, integrate, share, and find meaning from each experience. No matter what color pajamas I happen to be wearing.

Afterword: One Year Later

Healing is a habit

As I finish writing this manuscript, it's been about one year since I left behind the warm, fragrant, and inspiring grounds of the Kerala hospital. My panchakarma experience left imprints on me, but as I've experienced after other retreats, the real work begins back home.

First, I was eager to share my experience with friends and family upon returning. I didn't have a Nine Perfect Strangers story to tell them, but I regaled them with the stories of my daily oiling, the beatings during massage, the delicious food, the walking, and the generous people I met. Most of all, I became a walking advertisement for panchakarma. I'd never felt, or looked, better—not through some drastic physical alteration, but through expressing my light spirit through my eyes, my voice, my pores.

Now, several relatives have since signed up for their own panchakarma, including my parents. They even gave an early draft of this manuscript to the doctors there. They all had as good a time as I did, and I even got to learn more about some of the treatments I didn't receive myself.

As I reflected in my writings at the hospital, leaning back into a mode of being taken care of wasn't easy for me. However, it did make it easy to live an Ayurvedic lifestyle there. At home, where I had to be an adult again and take care of myself, I did my best to hold onto the rituals and practices that suited my constitution.

I couldn't wear white pajamas daily, of course, but I adopted a kind of uniform for myself and became more open to wearing relaxed clothes on the weekends. I swapped my "health food" salads and smoothies, and large-portions of western-style food eaten late in the evening for cooked foods and lighter, earlier dinners. I drank ginger tea all the time, and my kitchen was stocked with aromatic Indian spices. I found myself craving my forty-five-minute self-guided stretching sessions, instead of intense workouts in the mornings.

And for a while, my body thrived—I had no digestive issues, I felt less stiff and sore in my muscles, my mind was clear and sharp, and I didn't catch any colds or flus for a whole year. I got small "tune ups" with Ayurvedic practitioners near me, and working with them was empowering. Because of my foundation, we were able to go into deep, specific protocols that weren't as extreme as panchakarma, but still quite effective.

Now at the one-year mark, though, I see myself slipping. My digestion is starting to weaken from a few too many cold or raw foods, and perhaps too much travel and changing environments, although I do now prioritize spending time in warmer climates.

While part of me initially sought panchakarma as another intense way to optimize my health, I now see it as part of my long-term health maintenance. A reminder to simplify. A reminder of how it feels to feel good in my body.

This book was inspired by a woman I went on a date with the night before I left Australia for my panchakarma. After panchakarma, instead of returning home to Portugal, I went back to Australia, to explore what I felt was a powerful romantic connection with that woman. We would go on to spend the entire year together and got engaged in December of that year. I hope to bring her for my next panchakarma, whenever or wherever it may happen to be.

Modern life can make it hard, if not impossible, to hold onto the values of simplicity and feeling good. I'm grateful I have Ayurveda as a north star of health when I get distracted by busyness and trends.

I have gratitude for my body's ability to handle everything I throw at it—and to release what it doesn't need when it is allowed to come home and rest. The Kerala hospital will always be that home for me, and Ayurveda a homecoming. But, until I return to that home, the feeling of wearing my white pajamas will always be with me.

Acknowledgements

To Martin, thank you for putting panchakarma on my radar, helping me navigate countless options, and encouraging me to go.

To the doctors, therapists, and medical staff, thank you for your utmost care, professionalism, and patience with my many questions about the treatments, Ayurveda medicine, and Kerala culture

To the chef, kitchen staff, and dining hall staff, thank you for nourishing my body so well, and inspiring me to incorporate Ayurvedic food principles into my lifestyle.

To the hospital housekeeping and cleaning staff, thank you for helping me feel comfortable, and keeping my space comfortable.

To the hospital grounds staff, thank you for maintaining a beautiful campus full of trees, plants, birds, and the like. The environment helped all of us heal, thanks to your work.

To the yoga teachers and temple priest, thank you for supporting my physical, mental, and spiritual growth during my stay.

To the other patients, my co-inmates, for those seventeen days, thank you for sharing more of yourselves and your journey with me. You opened my heart and helped me feel greater compassion for others.

To you, the reader, thank you for your interest in my experience. I hope you find inspiration, learning, and compassion through my words.

And finally, to my body. Thank you for accepting the medicine, in the form of treatments, concoctions, food, exercise, spiritual practices, and more. We did well together, and I promise to continue to love you, as you are, without expectation.

Thank you for taking the time to read *White Pajamas*. Online reviews are incredibly important for authors like me and readers like you. They help new readers discover books they'll love and encourage authors like me to continue writing.

If you enjoyed *White Pajamas*, please leave a review on Amazon. Scan the QR code below on your phone to easily and quickly leave a review.

About the author

Kunal Gupta is an entrepreneur, investor, and author known for his insightful and unique perspectives.

2034 is Kunal's debut in fiction, where he blends his understanding and curiosity about artificial intelligence with a visionary narrative about the future. His other books include his firsthand life experiences and lessons on personal growth, business, technology, mindfulness, and health, reflecting his passions and expertise.

Born, raised, and educated in Canada, Kunal studied software engineering from the University of Waterloo and artificial intelligence at the University of Oxford.

Kunal founded and successfully scaled an advertising technology company, serving as Chief Everything Officer for 15 years. Based in New York at the time, he had the opportunity to see the world, collaborating with teams and clients across 30+ countries.

Deeply committed to mindfulness and mental health, he integrates these principles into his everyday life and enjoys sharing them with those around him regularly.

Engage with Kunal live at **kunalgpt.com**
Follow his blog and newsletter at **howto.live**
Discover more about his journey at **kunalgupta.live**

Kunal is donating 100% of book proceeds to charities promoting AI literacy and education.

Printed in Dunstable, United Kingdom